POSTNATAL
EXERCISES

Also available from Century

The Breastfeeding Book Máire Messenger
Exercises for Childbirth Barbara Dale and Johanna Roeber
Twins Averil Clegg and Anne Woollett
Toddler Taming Dr Christopher Green
The Right Food for your Kids Louise Templeton
Baby Play Dr Pat Petrie

POSTNATAL EXERCISES

A six-month fitness programme for mother and baby

Barbara Whiteford & Margie Polden

Foreword by George Pinker CVO, FRCS, FRCOG

Photographs by Sandra Lousada

CENTURY
LONDON · MELBOURNE · AUCKLAND · JOHANNESBURG

Postnatal Exercises: A six-month fitness programme for mother and baby was conceived, edited and designed by Frances Lincoln Limited, Apollo Works, 5 Charlton Kings Road, London NW5 2SB

Medical consultant Dr David Harvey

First published in Great Britain in 1984 by
Century Hutchinson Ltd
Brookmount House, 62-65 Chandos Place
Covent Garden, London WC2N 4NW

Reprinted 1985, 1987
Revised edition 1988

Century Hutchinson Australia Pty Ltd
PO Box 496, 16-22 Church Street
Hawthorn, Victoria 3122, Australia

Century Hutchinson New Zealand Ltd
PO Box 40-086, Glenfield
Auckland 10, New Zealand

Century Hutchinson South Africa Pty Ltd
PO Box 337, Bergvlei 2012, South Africa

British Library Cataloguing in Publication Data
Whiteford, Barbara
    Postnatal exercises.
    1. Physical fitness for women   2. Postnatal care
    I. Title   II. Polden, Margie
    613.7'045   RA781

ISBN 0 7126 2464 3

Printed in Hong Kong

CONTENTS

FOREWORD

The importance of rest and planned exercises in the days and weeks after the birth of your baby cannot be too strongly emphasized. It is a time when the body is recuperating and adjusting to a new way of life. It is therefore particularly helpful to women to have such a book which sensitively and sensibly informs mothers of what can be done to obtain the best result for themselves and their baby and to avoid some of the disabilities which follow childbirth without care.

The text is written from experience in every sense and this gives the advice and understanding which women will find helpful and easy to follow. The chapters on the emotional factors following pregnancy, care of the baby and handling of the baby and the particular attention paid to problems relating to posture and back pain following childbirth are valuable additions to the very important physiotherapy advice on how to regain a healthy physique after the baby. The authors are well known for the enormous help which they have given to mothers in their practical care over the years. It is excellent that their advice is now available to all mothers for guidance in preparing for a time which is often neglected, the return to health and normal physical well-being after the baby. The illustrations greatly add to the text and the authors are to be complimented on the compilation of this book.

George Pinker CVO, FRCS, FRCOG

INTRODUCTION

The drama of birth is the climax of nine long months of waiting and preparation for all mothers. Lying there with your baby, you may feel new energy, relief and euphoria, or perhaps you just feel exhausted, homesick and sore. You might have been prepared by your antenatal classes, books you have read or the experience of friends for the wide-ranging and abnormal intensity of moods which are an inevitable part of becoming a parent. However, you may have thought that after your baby was born, at least your body would return to normal straight away. You remember yourself as you were before pregnancy – firm and upright. You watched with pride your blooming, expanding abdomen and breasts as pregnancy advanced, but now the birth is over you expected to find yourself back as you were. Instead you are faced with a third stage – flabby, slouching and droopy, a woman whom you barely recognize.

Although you may only just be beginning to realize how much has to be done for your small, utterly dependent baby, you also know that you will need to do something positive for yourself to return to the way you were. For nine months your body was adapting to carry the growing baby; fortunately it does not take nearly as long to restore it to normal. Some of the changes occur within hours of your baby's birth: the uterus starts contracting down immediately, returning to its normal size by about six weeks; you will also lose a large amount of fluid in the days immediately following delivery. Even so, your muscles will still look, feel and be slack, stretched and weak. How quickly these return to normal appearance and function will depend a little on nature, but mostly on you.

Using the exercises

The exercises in this book are carefully graded to suit you from immediately after the birth right up to six months later, when your body is strong again. They are suitable for you regardless of your age, shape, current fitness and type of labour. (If you are in the least worried about your health, do discuss this with your

family doctor before starting the more strenuous exercises, especially if you have had a previous history of back problems.)
The subdivision into three sections (0-6 weeks, 6 weeks to 3 months, 3-6 months) only offers a rough guide and is designed for the normal woman and her rate of progress. If, for example, you are an older mother, or perhaps one who has had a Caesarean section, or if you took very little exercise prior to and during your pregnancy, then you will need to spend longer on the early exercises, perfecting them before moving on to the next stage. On the other hand, if you are a young mother who exercised regularly right up to your normal delivery, then you may feel able to advance to the second and then third stages a week or so earlier than suggested. Some useful ways of testing the strength of your important muscles (see pages 52 and 99) are included to help you assess your progress. Remember, too, that even if you did not feel like starting your exercises immediately, or even weeks after the birth, it is never too late to start.

Arranging your exercise schedule

If this is your first baby you may be surprised just how totally absorbing, and possibly frustrating, you find your new role. You cannot hear a baby's cry without assuming that it must be yours; you cannot go out for more than a few minutes for fear that you will be needed and you strongly believe that no-one else can comfort your baby. All these feelings are normal and natural and are probably there to ensure that women will satisfy their babies' many needs. It follows, therefore, that any programme of exercises must not force you into unwanted and uncomfortable separation from your baby, so most of the exercises in this book are designed to be done at home or anywhere that is convenient and comfortable.

Helping your baby's development

Alongside your own exercises, there are recommended positions, handling and play for your baby at the relevant stages of development. Just as in labour, when your knowledge enables you to direct your energy to coping with the contractions, if you are informed and confident in the handling of your baby, you will be more relaxed and fulfilled as a mother, and your baby will feel more secure and thus more contented in your care.

Rest and relaxation

Rest and relaxation are as vital as exercise in the early stages after birth, so it is important at the start of your exercise programme to be sensible and flexible about it. If you have been up all night and feel exhausted, then postpone the exercises until you have had a rest. If you feel energetic, repeat the appropriate exercises a few more times; but take care not to overdo them as you will do more harm than good if you strain your muscles or overtire yourself. Observe your body rhythms and do not believe that an exercise must hurt to be beneficial. On the contrary, exercises should feel comfortable and make you feel good. Bear in mind that you have just been through one of the most exhausting and strenuous events of your life.

YOUR BODY BEFORE AND AFTER THE BIRTH

During pregnancy, you have undergone gradual changes to your physique, posture and emotions, yet within a matter of hours you have produced your baby and have started to experience a whole new range of changes. Some begin restoring your body to its former state, and others help you provide the necessary love, food and care for your baby.

The physical changes that take place are quite dramatic: naturally it does not take as long for the body to return to its pre-pregnancy state as it does to nurture a developing fetus from a single cell to an eight pound baby. In order to understand these postnatal physical changes and to see where exercise can help, it is helpful to familiarize yourself with your anatomy and to look at the way it is affected by both pregnancy and birth.

The pelvic girdle The pelvic girdle is the bony framework at the bottom of your body. It is made up of four sets of bones; the first and most obvious are the big hip bones, which join in front at the symphysis pubis. They curve upwards to form two bony wings just beneath your waist and downwards to give you the bones you sit on. Wedged between these at the back is the sacrum, (the base of the spine) joined to the hip bones at the sacro-iliac joints. Finally there is the coccyx, all that remains of the human tail.

Like all the other joints of the body the pelvic joints are held together by ligaments. Normally little or no movement takes place in the pelvic joints, but during pregnancy, special tissue-softening hormones lead to the gradual softening and stretching of the body's ligaments which enable both the entrance and exit of the pelvis to increase in size as your baby passes through during labour.

Curving between the sacrum and the head are the twenty-four bones of the spine. If you put one hand on your symphysis pubis, and the other on your sacrum, you will see that the distance from back to front is not very great; in fact the internal diameter of the pelvis from back to front is only 10-12 cm (4-5 in). Usually

The pelvic girdle

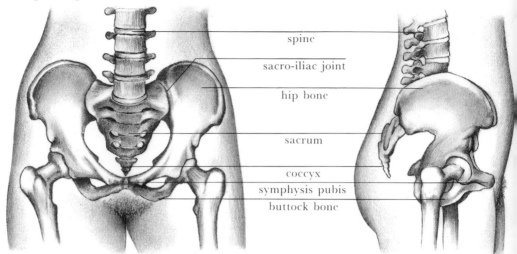

spine

sacro-iliac joint

hip bone

sacrum

coccyx

symphysis pubis

buttock bone

your pelvic organs – bladder, uterus and rectum – fit quite comfortably into this space, but by the end of your pregnancy the baby in the uterus makes things a very tight squeeze.

The ligaments

Ligaments are inelastic bands of supportive tissue which help hold your joints together. During pregnancy the ligaments soften and stretch due to the influence of the hormones progesterone and relaxin, resulting in some relaxation in all the joints, not just the pelvic girdle. The effects of these changes can persist for up to five months after your baby is born, and may be felt as aching or sometimes pain, especially in the joints of your back, the joints between your spine and pelvis (the sacro-iliac joints) and occasionally radiating into your buttock or leg. The joint in the front of your pelvis (the symphysis pubis) can give rise to problems as well.

The uterus

The uterus is a muscular bag which normally weighs less than 100g (3.5 oz), and fits snugly into your pelvic girdle along with the other organs. By the end of your pregnancy the uterus alone weighs about 1 kg (2.2 lb).

Involution

Immediately after the birth your uterus can be felt through your soft abdominal wall just below the umbilicus. It is about the size it was at the fourth month of pregnancy. It starts to contract down straight away – the process known as involution – returning to its former size and position by six weeks. The contractions of involution may initially be felt as 'after pains', which will be more pronounced if you already have one or more children. Breastfeeding stimulates these contractions, which may feel like period pains or the discomfort felt in very early labour. Involution is entirely involuntary; it is a normal part of the reproductive process. (See page 49 for further help.)

The blood forced out by your contracting uterus from the raw

The pelvic organs

  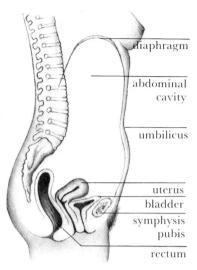

diaphragm

abdominal cavity

umbilicus

uterus
bladder
symphysis pubis

rectum

At the end of pregnancy
Because of your bulging abdomen your posture alters, and the organs are compressed.

Immediately after the birth
You will probably still look about 6 months pregnant.

6 weeks after the birth
Your uterus should have contracted down to its normal shape, size and position.

site of the placenta is called the lochia. It should be red for the first few days, gradually changing to brown, then yellow, and finally disappearing between two to six weeks. You should report any large clots, sudden heavy loss or offensive smell to your doctor, midwife or health visitor.

Within about two weeks of the delivery it should no longer be possible to feel your uterus in your abdomen, as it has shrunk down into your pelvis (though it is still larger than normal). When you go for your postnatal check your doctor will examine you to make sure your uterus has fully contracted.

The pelvic floor

Holding everything in place underneath the pelvis is a hammock of muscle known as the pelvic floor, which is enormously stretched by childbirth. The pelvic floor muscles are divided into a deep and a superficial layer and have three openings: the urethra (from the bladder); the vagina (from the uterus); and the rectum and anus (from the bowel). The muscle fibres surround each of these openings in a figure of eight, the front part looping round the vagina and urethra and the back part around the anus. The muscles are interconnected and work as one complete unit. Some of the muscle fibres are able to work strongly over long periods, while others can only work in short bursts (slow or fast twitch fibres, page 52). The wedge of muscles between the vagina and the anus is known as the perineum. If you have an episiotomy to assist the safe delivery of your baby, this is where it will be.

The muscles making up the pelvic floor are quite small; they are held together by sheets of non-stretchy tissue called fascia. Before pregnancy most women are completely unaware of them, yet they are very important for health and comfort as they support the pelvic organs and prevent the bladder and bowel from leaking. (Strong pelvic floor muscles are also essential for a successful sex life.)

During pregnancy the pelvic floor will have had to carry the increased weight of your baby and uterus; during the second

The pelvic floor muscles

clitoris

urethra

vagina

perineal area

anus

possible
episiotomy
sites

stage of labour it will have thinned out and stretched open around your baby's head and body. It may also have been damaged by an episiotomy or a tear, and many women experience acute pain in this area for several days.

If you have had stitches following a large tear or episiotomy, you may need to take mild pain-killers for a while. The wound should be kept as clean and dry as possible by frequent bathing and changing of sanitary towels. Your obstetric physiotherapist may use ultrasound or pulsed short wave to promote healing and relieve pain. She may also show you how to use ice and heat – two to three minutes' massage with an ice cube or five to ten minutes' gentle warmth with a hair dryer (set at its lowest heat), or with a reading lamp, can be soothing and give relief from the pain and can be continued at home.

If you have had an episiotomy or tear it may help you overcome any anxieties you have about it if you look at it in a mirror after a few days. You will probably be surprised how well bonded the wound looks. Remember the more often you contract your pelvic floor muscles, the quicker their recovery will be.

Three common problems

1 Sitting down Occasionally the post-delivery pain is so severe that some women are forced to feed their babies standing up! Sitting on a rubber ring or two folded pillows with a gap between them can prove helpful by removing pressure from the area. Make sure you put the part of you that is sorest in the hole in the middle.

2 Coughing, sneezing or laughing As you cough a lot of pressure is exerted on your stitches, and it can feel as if they are bursting. It is much more comfortable if you remember to squeeze in and lift your pelvic floor muscles while you cough, sneeze, blow your nose or laugh (see page 52).

3 Bowel movements You will *not* tear your stitches if you have to strain to open your bowels. Support them with a folded sanitary towel to control the pain (see page 16).

If discomfort and pain in this area persist when you walk, sit, stand or make love, be sure to mention it to your doctor when you have your postnatal check. If scar tissue is causing problems, therapeutic ultrasound can be administered by a physiotherapist to soften it.

Sexual problems

There is no 'normal' time to resume sexual intercourse, although most women prefer to wait until the lochia is finished. You may feel desire as early as seven days or not until seven months after your baby's birth (or even longer)!

When you do both feel like trying intercourse, but you find it is very painful, stop and leave it for a few days. It may be that using a lubricating gel (obtainable from any chemist) would help your partner achieve a gentler penetration, or that adopting another position would make a difference to pain in your vagina and breasts. If you both lie on your sides or you lie or sit above your partner, then you will be able to control his penetration and the pressure on your tender breasts.

Sex is not just a matter of physical comfort, of course, and you may find that your feelings towards your partner seem to change after the birth (see page 35). Guilt about this apparent change, fear of pain or damage to the perineum, anxiety about becoming pregnant again, or simply preoccupation with your baby can all affect your desire for sex. You may also feel flabby and unattractive. It is far better to talk these things through with your partner rather than maintain a martyred silence. After all, there are many other ways of reaching mutual satisfaction apart from actual intercourse.

If you are concerned that intercourse will be painful or impossible, when you go for your postnatal check at about six weeks, do not be afraid to mention it. (This is also the time to discuss contraception if you have not done so already.) Your perineum and vagina should be checked for healing and the presence of infection, the strength of your vaginal muscles tested, and your cervix examined to exclude the presence of a cervical erosion (ulcer) which could be a cause of pain during lovemaking. If your vaginal opening is found to be too tight, it can be treated – perhaps by gentle stretching. If you find that, far from a vagina which is too tight, you have been left feeling loose and floppy so that neither of you gets any pleasure from intercourse, you should also mention this. It may be that an intensive regime of pelvic floor exercises will cure this, but if not, then a minor surgical repair may be recommended to correct the problem.

Stress incontinence

Stress incontinence may have troubled you at the end of your pregnancy; more likely it is something which only developed after your baby was born. It is the uncontrollable leakage of urine from your bladder when you cough, sneeze, laugh or blow your nose, when you pick up something heavy, or perhaps run for a bus. Your pelvic floor exercise (see page 52) can be the answer to this problem. Practise this little tightening movement constantly: once a day is *not* enough. You should aim at four good contractions every 15 minutes or so. Initially you may have very poor sensation around the vagina but it should gradually return to normal and you will be able to feel these muscles working together, lifting inwards and upwards. Use the pelvic floor contraction while coughing or blowing your nose. As you breathe in to cough, quickly draw the pelvic floor in and up; hold it tightly braced until the cough is over, and only then relax.

Although stress incontinence is usually cured by correct and conscientious exercising, sometimes you may have such badly stretched internal ligaments or vaginal and urethral tissue that a small 'repair' operation could be necessary. If after three months of honest exercising you are still leaking embarrassingly, return to your doctor for further help. If a repair is indicated, your gynaecologist may prefer to wait until your family is complete before performing the operation.

Haemorrhoids

Haemorrhoids, or piles, are swollen varicose veins in your rectum and anus. Sometimes they appear in pregnancy, sometimes only after the baby is born – pushing in the second stage of labour can make them worse and they can be extremely painful, making sitting down well nigh impossible. (Ask for a rubber ring if this is the case.) Once again, your pelvic floor exercise will help by improving the circulation in this sensitive area and therefore reducing the pain. A crushed ice-pack gently applied to the grape-like swelling can also give relief, and there are anaesthetic ointments which your doctor can prescribe. Haemorrhoids usually resolve after a short while.

The abdominal muscles

The first thing many mothers do after their delivery is to touch their stomachs and notice how flat they feel, yet how flabby. This is because the abdominal muscles which have been stretched round the uterus do not of course immediately return to their original shape – and will not properly without help.

The muscle layers

The abdominal corset, as it is known, consists of four layers of muscles. There are two superficial muscles – the recti abdominis – running straight up and down; two pairs of oblique muscles; and one pair of transverse muscles. This abdominal corset joins down the mid-line, where a strip of fibrous tissue called the linea alba – normally about 1 cm (½ in) wide – can actually be seen on thin, muscular people. The abdominal muscles are weakest in the front, where the recti abdominis are only one layer deep. The other muscles overlap to form three layers at the sides.

How the muscles stretch

During pregnancy the abdominal muscles stretch around the growing uterus; a woman who normally measures about 33 cm (13 in) from breastbone to pubis can stretch to around 50 cm (20

Changes in the abdominal muscles

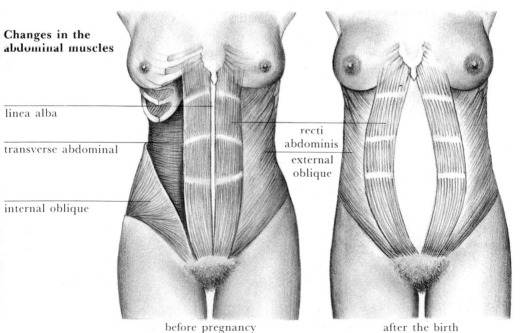

linea alba

transverse abdominal

internal oblique

recti abdominis

external oblique

before pregnancy   after the birth

in), while her waist might increase from 66 cm (26 in) to 101 cm (46 in)! As the body's ligaments soften during pregnancy, the linea alba also softens; in late pregnancy it is quite common for the two recti to separate above and below the umbilicus. Unless they are very thin, few women realize this is happening because this condition – known as diastasis recti – is completely painless. However, separation weakens the abdominal wall, which could give rise to constant backache. It may seem strange that back pain can be brought about by weak front muscles, but that is the case; apart from holding your abdominal organs in place and giving you a waistline, the abdominal muscles also support the back. That is why it is vitally important to begin the programme of exercises as soon as possible after the birth, to bring the abdominal muscles back to their former strength and tautness, so that you avoid difficulties with backache.

Multiple births

If you are carrying more than one baby you will inevitably feel more tired and uncomfortable towards the end of your pregnancy. Postnatally your abdominal muscles will be much weaker and the separation between the recti will be much greater, so that it probably will take much longer to reach full recovery. A new mother with only one baby often finds that 6 to 8 weeks pass before she has time to devote to stengthening weak muscles; mothers of two or even more new babies will invariably be too tired and busy for regular exercising until perhaps four or more months have passed. You will probably have to spend more time than mothers of single babies on the early stages of the exercise programme, and be particularly careful not to increase fatigue by trying to do too much too soon. No matter how long it is before you are able to start, you should be aware that it is *never too late*.

Constipation

Some women suffer from constipation during pregnancy, while others become constipated following the birth of their babies. Some iron pills and pain-killers are constipating and the hormones of pregnancy, which soften your ligaments, also relax your intestines so that they are not as efficient as they used to be at expelling their contents. Once your baby is born an additional factor comes into play – your abdominal muscles are now loose and floppy and give very poor support to the intestines and bowel.

Another cause of postnatal constipation is simply fear of straining or tearing stitches in the perineum. If this is the case, support your stitches with a clean sanitary towel as you bear down to open your bowels.

If you are constipated it is very important to eat extra high-fibre foods, such as wholemeal bread, bran cereals, fresh fruit (do not peel your apples and pears), celery, cabbage and so on. You can add bran to your soups, stewed fruit, or yoghurt – and be sure to drink extra fluid too. If, in spite of a sensible diet, you are still in trouble, ask your doctor to recommend a suitable laxative – you should not take anything which might affect your baby if you are breastfeeding.

Structure of the breasts

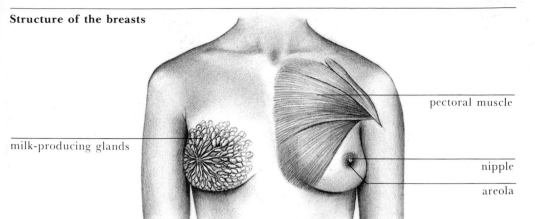

milk-producing glands

pectoral muscle

nipple

areola

The breasts

The breasts are neither muscle nor ligament; they are mainly fat with a small amount of glandular tissue. During pregnancy they will have enlarged so that your bra size may have increased substantially. By the end of your pregnancy some of the fat under the skin of the breasts will have been absorbed and the milk producing glands will have grown and developed and you may have noticed the first few drops of colostrum – the substance that precedes true breast milk – being secreted.

Production of milk

After your baby is delivered the changing hormones stimulate your breasts to produce milk. True milk does not 'come in' until around the third day and until then the breasts continue to produce protein-rich colostrum. As the breasts fill with milk they become firm, large and heavy, and as your baby feeds or you express the milk yourself, a further supply will be stimulated. Within a few weeks the supply and your baby's demands will probably have coincided.

Around three to five days after the birth, the breasts may become hard, pink, hot and tender – this is called engorgement. It may be necessary to express a little milk first to soften the area around the nipple (the areola) so that the baby can suck properly. Your doctor or midwife will advise you on how best to relieve the problem, which seldom lasts more than a day or two.

If you are breastfeeding it is usually thought to be important to wear a well-supporting bra as the extra weight in your breasts may cause them to sag. Unlike muscle, breast tissue does not recover once stretched. However, although there are no exercises for the breasts themselves, it is certainly possible to improve the strength of the pectorals, their supporting muscles.

Chest toning exercises (see page 60) will not prevent your breasts from drooping, but they will help improve your posture, which is probably the most important factor in determining the position of your breasts on the chest wall. If you stand or sit with rounded shoulders, your breasts are more likely to droop. Keep your back straight, lift your ribs and remember to keep your shoulders down and relaxed. Using the pectoral muscles vigorously will improve circulation and so may help lactation.

The muscles of the back, buttocks and thighs

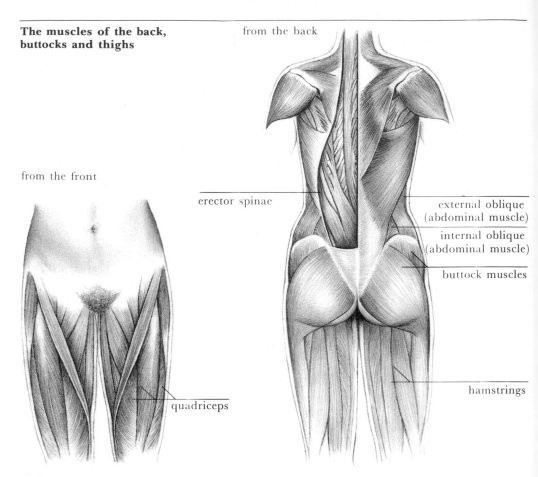

from the back

from the front

erector spinae

external oblique (abdominal muscle)

internal oblique (abdominal muscle)

buttock muscles

hamstrings

quadriceps

The back, buttocks and legs

After the birth, it is extremely important to strengthen back, buttock and leg muscles, as any weakness in these areas may lead to poor posture, bad lifting techniques and eventual backache. This is so important that a whole chapter has been devoted to it (see page 22).

Your legs may have become heavier in pregnancy, especially if you suffered from oedema (fluid retention). However, not all this swelling can be attributed to fluid – some of it will be fat. Using and exercising your leg muscles will also improve the circulation and lessen the swelling.

Weight loss

After delivery you will have lost the weight of your baby, the amniotic fluid, and the placenta – probably about 3-5kg (7-11 lb). You may lose an extra 1-1½ kg (2-3 lb) over the next few days as you excrete excess fluid from both tissues and extra blood volume. The uterus gradually shrinks from 1 kg (2.2 lb) to about 50-70 g (2-3 oz) during the next six weeks. However, you will probably find you are still heavier than you were before you became pregnant – maybe considerably so. This difference in weight is made up of fat.

Diet

If you are breastfeeding, some of this fat may be broken down to help produce breast milk and you may also be burning much of it up simply by doing the endless jobs involved in being a mother. However, just as it was during pregnancy, it is a myth that if you are breastfeeding you must eat for two. Dieticians advise that a breastfeeding mother only needs about 200-500 calories more than one who is bottlefeeding. Pay attention to the quality of your food, as well as the quantity, avoiding the 'empty calories' contained in sweets, cakes and biscuits. A well-balanced diet (including protein foods, such as meat and fish or beans and other legumes, dairy foods, fruit, vegetables, fibre and limited carbohydrate) is vital for an adequate supply of breast milk. Always be careful about the amount of fat in your diet — butter, margarine, cheese, cream, fat meat, oils and fried foods. Skimmed milk will give you all the nutrients you need with half the calories. You may find you are very thirsty, so take extra fluid, but if you are overweight remember that nearly all drinks except water contain calories.

If you are still over your ideal weight by the time your baby is about six months old, then adjust the quantity of your food intake while maintaining its quality and balance. Record your weight regularly (but not more than once a week) to ensure you are gradually losing your excess fat. If you are breastfeeding, do not attempt any crash diets as they may affect your health, energy and milk supply. However, there is nothing to restrict the bottlefeeding mother from dieting sensibly from the start. If, despite adequate diet and rest, you feel excessively tired and irritable, you may be anaemic and iron supplements may be prescribed by your doctor.

Obesity

You may be one of those women who finds herself still in her maternity clothes months after her baby was born. You hear conflicting advice from well-meaning friends and relatives about diet; you don't want to affect your ability to breastfeed but you worry that your partner will no longer find you attractive if you do not lose weight soon. Sometimes you find yourself so miserable that you eat to console yourself, though you know that this is only making the problem worse.

It is important not to let your problem become an obsession which can be far worse than the weight itself. Your first step should be to seek expert advice: go to your doctor and ask for a referral to a dietician. She will take your individual circumstances into consideration — your weight before pregnancy, your energy requirements, whether you are breastfeeding or not, your budget — and then advise you on what you can eat to lose weight safely and with certainty.

Secondly, try to borrow or buy some clothes that are loose fitting and comfortable, but which are not maternity clothes, so you are not mistakenly asked 'When is it due?'. Thirdly, remember that your partner has always found more than just your body attractive. His greatest wish will be to see you well and happy so that he can enjoy his new family.

POSTURE AND BACK CARE

Your posture

Your posture is the way you hold your body; it can often tell the world how you feel. Everyone makes assumptions about people based on their posture – good posture is as important as a smile or an easy manner.

What is good posture? It is not only a matter of appearance but also of function – it should be efficient, comfortable and adaptable to the movements and positions used throughout the day. It is largely controlled by a reflex (subconscious) mechanism but is also considerably influenced by outside factors, such as emotions, neglected or damaged muscles and weight change. In pregnancy it is also affected by the softening of ligaments and the resulting joint laxity. Fortunately most postural faults can be corrected in a young, healthy person, but if they are not, they may go on to produce joint changes, sometimes leading to arthritis and long-standing discomfort.

How pregnancy influences posture

During your pregnancy three main factors contribute to the adjustment (and often deterioration) of your posture. The first is the hormonal influence, causing your ligaments to soften; the second is the gradual increase and changed distribution of your weight; the third is your self image and emotions – your feelings about your shape and the developing baby. Unless you are aware of these gradual changes you may find that after your baby is born, you still look several months pregnant. Your body's postural reflex has over-compensated and may be 'stuck' in the stance of pregnancy. You will need to re-educate your muscles to correct it.

Assessing your posture

To help you assess your posture, you will need to be aware of the common postural problems of the pregnant woman. As the baby grows in her uterus, a combination of the forward movement of her centre of gravity and stretched, weak abdominal muscles cause her to adapt by hollowing her lower spine, pushing her knees back, rounding her shoulders and poking her chin forward. Her softened ligaments allow an unusual flexibility of

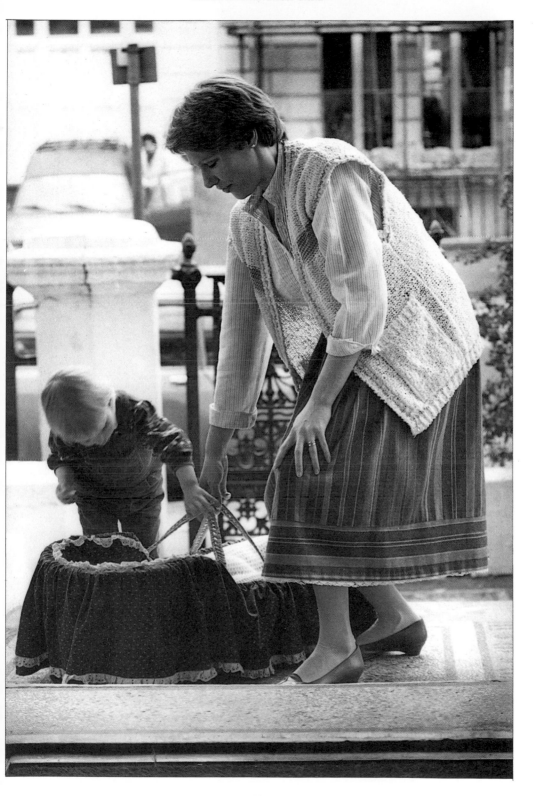

the spine, and if she is not aware that her posture is faulty, her back muscles eventually shorten as her abdominal muscles stretch, with extra stresses placed on the ligaments and bones of the spine and pelvis. The usual result is backache.

After the birth, your perineal stitches (or in the case of a Cacsarcan section, abdominal stitches) may be so uncomfortable when you first get up to walk that your whole body sags forward and you shuffle along anxiously with your legs together. Holding an abnormal position because of pain, or the fear of it, is very tiring. You can be certain that your stitches are safe and that 'standing tall' as described below, and taking a gentle walk, will improve not only your posture and appearance, but also your circulation and comfort.

Correcting your posture

1 Look at yourself sideways in a long mirror, or ask a friend to check you. Stand as tall as you can: imagine someone has grabbed a tuft of hair from the top of your head and is pulling it upwards.
2 Tuck your buttocks under and pull in your abdominal muscles as you tilt your whole pelvis backwards (your pubic bone should move forwards and up as this happens).
3 Move your feet about 30 cm (12 in) apart and feel the weight on their outside edges.
4 Take a deep breath and expand your ribs upwards and outwards, arms hanging loosely but rolled slightly outwards.

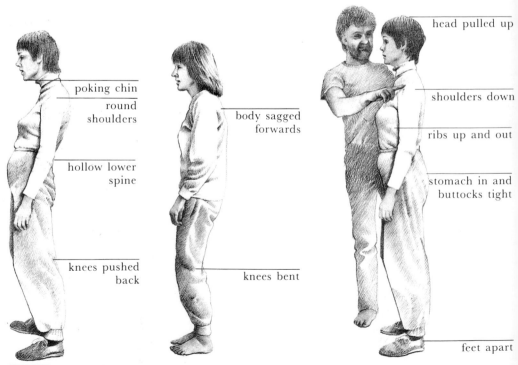

poking chin
round shoulders

body sagged forwards

head pulled up

shoulders down

ribs up and out

hollow lower spine

stomach in and buttocks tight

knees pushed back

knees bent

feet apart

Two examples of poor posture after birth   **Corrected posture**

5 Now relax your breathing to a slow, deep rhythm that is natural to you.

Feel your new posture; note the muscles that are working to hold it for you, especially your abdominal and buttock muscles. It may feel odd and unnatural at first, but be reassured by your mirror image or your critical friend that it has now improved.

Try to visualize that your muscles are made of a special type of elastic which has been overstretched but which, with use, has the power to rejuvenate. Now feel the muscles you are using to maintain your new, corrected posture, and see if you can continue to hold it for as long as possible throughout the day while you stand, sit or walk. At first this will be a conscious effort, but gradually the muscles themselves will adapt by becoming shorter and more elastic, and you will no longer need to think about them as they hold your improved position. Try to introduce your new awareness of good posture into everything you do, whether it is working or resting. As well as your baby, of course, it could be one of the long-term benefits of childbirth.

Other ways to improve your posture

1 When you sit down in a chair to feed your baby or to relax, make sure you choose one that is the right height and depth, and which gives good support. The ideal chair is one with a firm back support into which you push your bottom, and a seat which provides support for your thighs while still allowing your knees to relax at right angles and your feet to rest flat on the floor. You may find it even more comfortable to put a cushion behind your waist. When you are feeding, lie your baby on a pillow on your lap and rest one or both feet on a footstool (or perhaps a pile of telephone directories or other large books). Both these aids will help raise your baby up towards your breasts, preventing the need to lean too far forward.

Good feeding position

Bad feeding position

2 When you lie down to rest, make sure you are comfortable and that your vulnerable back is not strained or twisted in any way. If you like to lie on your back, put a pillow under your thighs to help flatten the hollow in your spine.

Lying on your front is an excellent position for relieving the pain of perineal stitches, haemorrhoids and backache. Make certain you put one or even two pillows under your waist, so that your pelvis is raised and your back flattened. You will probably also find it more comfortable to have a pillow or two under your head and shoulders, so that your enlarged breasts are free from pressure. (If you have had a Caesarean section you will not be able to use this position immediately, but in two to three weeks you too will be able to enjoy it.) Rest in this position several times a day if you can. It has probably been impossible to lie on your stomach for months, so enjoy it now.

3 Shoes also have an important influence on your posture. Those with a 2½-5 cm (1-2 in) heel are ideal as they lessen the tendency to hollow the lower back. It is important not to wear very high heels too often, as they will throw your weight even further forward and exaggerate the curve of your spine.

Back care

Back problems are among the most common complaints of pregnancy and the postnatal period. As has already been described, during pregnancy hormones cause the ligaments of the pelvis and spine to soften and stretch, so that poor posture, faulty lifting, excessive weight gain or a previous back probem may then contribute to strain on the joints of the spine or pelvis, and cause backache or pain. The joint laxity caused by the softened ligaments may persist for five months after your baby is born, so extra care must be taken during this time. Refer to the earlier hints on good posture as well as those given opposite, and remember that the best treatment for back problems is prevention.

The sacro-iliac and lower back ligaments

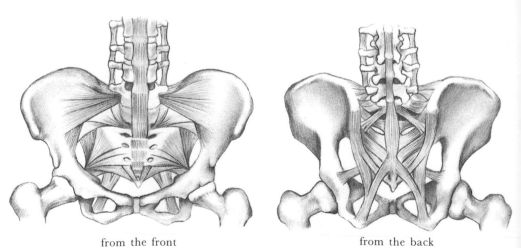

from the front   from the back

26

Preventing back damage

1 When you sit down, make sure your bottom is pressed well into the back of the chair; and perhaps use a pillow to hold your back upright.

Do not slump or slouch in a soft chair.

2 As you roll over or get out of bed, avoid twisting or turning with your knees apart. First tighten your abdominal muscles, bend your knees and roll onto your side; then push yourself up into the sitting position with your arms, swing both your legs over the bed, knees together, and stand up. Remember to reverse this when getting back into bed.

3 When you are standing to do household chores, put one foot up on a low stool or two or three telephone directories, or rest one foot on the bottom shelf of a cupboard, letting you use your back more comfortably.

4 When lifting a toddler or a heavy weight such as a bucket full of soaking nappies, pull your abdominal muscles in, tuck in your buttocks and brace your pelvic floor. Keeping your spine straight, bend your legs to kneel or squat down, bring the weight close to your body, and, using your stronger thighs to bear the weight, slowly rise to standing. This will protect the much smaller muscles and ligaments of your back, and is also, incidentally, an excellent way of toning flabby thigh muscles. If you are lifting your baby in a carry cot, have the head nearest to you – this will put less strain on your back. Never lift when bending or twisting to the side. When pushing or pulling a weight, such as moving furniture, make sure your knees are bent and mobile.

5 Remember to protect your back by doing low household chores, such as making the bed, bathing your baby or dressing your toddler, on your knees. Squat or kneel to pick things up off the floor.

6 If you are vacuuming or sweeping, move your weight forwards and backwards over your front leg, keeping your back straight; avoid the risky twisting movement while bending forward.

7 When choosing a sling, buggy or pram for carrying or transporting your baby, think of your back (see page 64). Choose a sling which carries your baby centrally (front or back) and which is adjustable so that you can raise your baby up so that his head rests on your breastbone. Choose a buggy or pram that has handles that are high enough – at least hip height – to push it without stooping forward.

8 Make sure the surface on which you change your baby is at the right height for you. About waist level is ideal in the early months, before your baby has learnt to roll. Then perhaps you can progress to changing him on the floor, sitting back on either heel with the other knee bent forward, foot flat on the floor with your baby as close to you as possible between your legs. Don't kneel down on both knees – this is as bad for your back as stooping over your baby.

9 If your bed is very soft, it will help if you slide a solid piece of block board between the mattress and the bed base, or put the mattress on the floor.

Coping with backache

In spite of your best endeavours, you may still find that backache is a problem in the postnatal period. Indeed many women experience it during pregnancy, beginning as early as the second month, but it usually does not last; if this happened to you, you may have assumed you would not be troubled again. When you noticed that first gnawing ache or twinge of pain after your baby was born, you sincerely hoped that it would pass, along with some of the other transient discomforts you have felt as a new mother. It may indeed go away, having been no more than a temporary irritation. On the other hand, it may persist, leaving you in intermittent or sometimes constant pain, so that you are practically immobilized, finding that you are unable to function normally until it passes.

Where backache occurs

By far the most common site of this ache or pain after birth is the sacro-iliac joint, where the spine joins the pelvis on either side. It is normally felt over the joint, (which lies immediately under one of the two dimples on either side of the spine), becoming acute on pressure or when twisting the lower spine. The pain may radiate into the whole buttock, and there is sometimes associated tenderness at the front over the pubic bone. The backache experienced can be constant, and there may be pain down the leg. Walking short distances is often reasonably comfortable, but the pain will then usually get progressively worse. It may be difficult to bear weight on the affected leg (such as when climbing stairs), there is little relief felt after lying down, and you may feel stiff after a period of sitting.

Intervertebral disc damage

Very severe pain may be caused by damage to a disc between the vertebrae of the spine, although this is unusual compared to backache due to the combination of softened ligaments, poor posture and excess weight. It may cause lumbago (incapacitating pain in the lower back) or sciatica (pain along the sciatic nerve – through the buttock, back of the thigh and calf and into the foot); the pain will be most severe when sitting, coughing and bending forwards – which will be restricted. Lying down usually relieves the symptoms. The treatment for disc problems is usually bed-rest. If this fails to help relieve your pain then see your doctor who may suggest a course of physiotherapy.

RELIEVING LOW BACK PAIN

Advice has already been given on how to protect your back, but if you experience persistent backache, there are several ways to alleviate and often cure sacro-iliac pain.

Try pelvic rocking, as described on page 84 under the exercise called 'Cat Arch'. If you are unable to kneel down on all fours when your back is aching, try the exercise while sitting or even standing up. If you experience back pain in bed, roll onto your side and, with your knees bent, rock your pelvis gently backwards and forwards. If this does not help, or if your pain is acute and stops you walking, then lie on the floor and try one or both of the following manoeuvres. Both help pain on either side; the first example illustrates relief for right-sided pain and the second for pain on the left.

KNEE TO SHOULDER PULLS
Bend your right leg up (as shown), holding it around the knee with your right hand, and with your left hand cupping the heel of the right foot, pull the right heel towards your groin. Keeping your shoulders flat and left leg straight, press the bent leg further up towards the right shoulder, as far as it will comfortably go. Slowly relax. Repeat several times, then, keeping your knees bent and together, roll onto your side, push up onto all fours, and stand carefully, keeping your back straight.

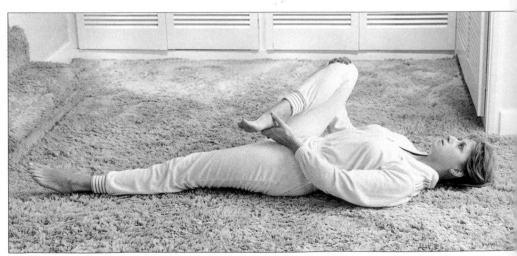

TWISTING ROCKS

Lie on your back on the floor. Bend your left leg and hook your toes under the outside of your right calf, rolling your left knee towards the right. Now take your right arm across your body so that your hand holds your left hip. Rock gently in this position; then roll back to the starting position. Relax slowly. Repeat several times. Again take care when you stand up – knees together to roll onto your side, then push onto all fours, and keep your back straight as you rise to stand.

Taking medical advice If your backache continues, as a first-aid measure try wearing a roll-on or pantie girdle to support the aching joints. It may give very good relief and will not weaken your abdominal muscles as long as you remember to use them to hold yourself in. If your backache begins to affect your ability to cope with your family, then do not hesitate to seek medical advice. Treatment may be as simple as one dramatic manipulation, or you may be advised very firmly to take a period of rest flat on your back. Whatever is needed, you must try to tackle the problem now, however inconvenient or impossible it may seem. Back problems have a habit of recurring as acute and crippling episodes or chronic, nagging aches.

YOUR FEELINGS
AFTER THE BIRTH

Emotional changes

No matter how intensely you looked forward to the birth of your baby, or how much you expected that the rewards of motherhood would compensate for your loss of freedom or job satisfaction, it is as well to be prepared for a tiring, tense and possibly traumatic first few weeks. Women change and develop emotionally as much as physically during the early days of motherhood.

In the same way that the enlarging uterus and softening ligaments of pregnancy trouble some women during the gestation of their babies – so the change in lifestyle from independence to motherhood can also prove painful for some. In fact, becoming a parent is one of life's most important revolutions, and is often described as a 'life crisis', similar to the upheaval involved in marriage, bereavement, changing or losing a job, or moving house. However, if you are prepared for some of the feelings and problems which can occur after your baby is born you may be able to cope with them more easily.

Immediate feelings after the birth

The way you feel in the first few hours following delivery can vary enormously. You may be euphoric, flat, detached, tearful, overjoyed, or disappointed. A lot will depend on the length and type of labour you have just experienced. Naturally you are going to feel more tired if your labour has been long and painful, especially if you missed out on more than one night's sleep. You may have set yourself all sorts of goals to achieve in labour, and feel a failure because, instead of an active, natural childbirth you ended up with pethidine, an epidural, an episiotomy and a forceps delivery. You may have set your heart on a golden haired daughter and have got instead a dark haired son with forceps marks on his face, who looks very much like your least favourite relation. Some women fall in love with their babies instantly, but many others have a detached feeling about them – their overriding reaction being a desire to roll over and go to sleep.

Apart from the initial fatigue that follows labour, tremendous changes in the hormonal balance may also affect the emotions.

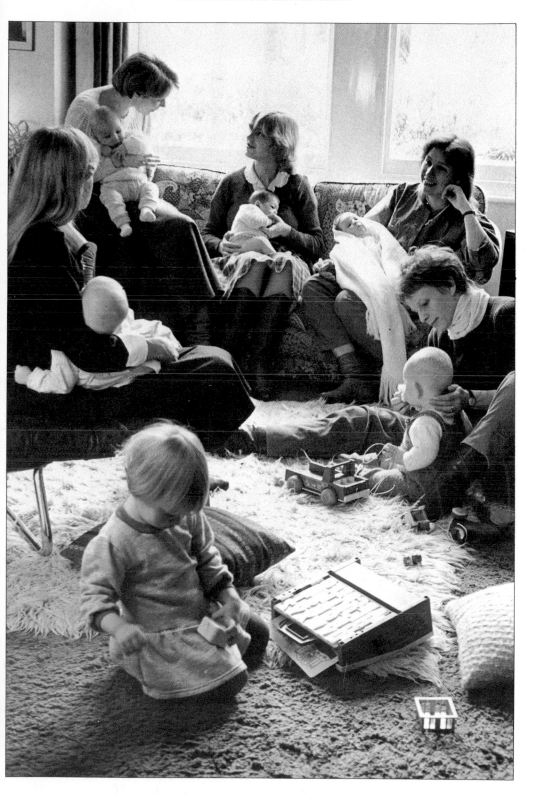

The hormones which have been controlling the pregnancy are replaced by those which stimulate the breasts to produce milk, and return the body to its pre-pregnant state. These changes may cause overwhelming shifts in mood.

Something you may not have been expecting is missing the presence of your baby within your body. Even though you have been longing for your balloon-like shape to disappear, you may feel empty and lonely after your baby is born and miss his movements intensely. (Your baby will almost certainly feel lonely too.) Another strange and probably completely unexpected feeling is a sense of anticlimax. Labour, which is often seen as the 'grand finale' of pregnancy before you return to normal, is actually the 'overture' to a completely new lifestyle.

'Baby blues'

'Baby blues' can be another distressing reaction. They usually creep up on you between two days and a week after the birth, or even later. Emotions that go up have to come down. If the first 48 hours of your role as mother has floated by in a haze of pink cloud, it can be a shock then to experience tearfulness, depression and feelings of helplessness. Little things may trigger bouts of crying – maybe your partner arrives five minutes late for visiting time; or a nurse speaks to you abruptly. You may also notice violent mood swings, one minute feeling intense surges of mother love, the next being driven to desperation because the baby is crying. The blues may simply overwhelm you because you hate hospital routines, your bed is uncomfortable, the food tasteless, your stitches hurt, and you feel homesick.

Early days at home

Once you are home with your baby the most devastating discovery for the first-time mother may be that you are on duty 24 hours a day, seven days a week – there is no let up. First-timers have the additional burden of having to learn how to be mothers and fathers – parents having a second or subsequent baby have learnt this lesson and birth is probably not such an overwhelming experience.

Many women who had responsible jobs feel failures because they cannot cope domestically – the chores pile up and they are still in their dressing-gowns by mid-afternoon. Breastfeeding and bottlefeeding both present problems, although you are more likely to feel a failure if you cannot breastfeed.

Catching up with sleep

Most young women are used to an uninterrupted night's sleep of eight to nine hours, and it can take several months until they get used to their new way of life and for the intense fatigue to disappear. Your motto at first should be, 'sleep when the baby sleeps', which is easy after a first baby, but not quite so easy if you already have older children. If you cannot fit in an hour or two's sleep during the day, make the most of little 'cat naps' whenever you can. Rest and relax – using the simple relaxation drill on page 40, and make sure that feeding times are restful and relaxing too: put your feet up or curl up on your side on your bed. Make up your mind that for a while you do not need a spotlessly clean house; this is something that your partner can help with. If cooking is a problem for both of you, convenience foods or take-away meals are worth the extra expense for a while.

Finally there will be days when rest is more important to you than exercises. Don't worry if you are unable to fit the exercises in every day, and don't exercise at 11.30 at night when you are dropping with fatigue.

Crisis measure

If you feel that you are so drained of energy you cannot go on any longer, a useful tip is to go to bed as soon as you have eaten supper – say at 7 pm – and sleep until your baby wakes for a feed. Ask your partner to bring the baby to you in bed; let him change the nappy – if necessary – half-way through the feed; then, when your baby is full of food and drops off to sleep, snuggle back into your covers and do the same, until the next feed.

Anxiety and stress

Anxiety is an emotion which may constantly plague you during those early weeks – feeding, changing, sleeping all seem fraught with uncertainties. You may reach the stage when you feel compelled to telephone your partner begging him to come home and relieve you. He is your link with the outside world and you need his support. Some parents try to continue their lives as if nothing had happened, determined that the baby should in no way alter their cosy twosome – but it is practically impossible initially to be a perfect mother, partner and lover simultaneously.

Your relationship with your partner

First time childbirth often disrupts a marriage in a way which can be totally unexpected – after all, a twosome which increases by 50 per cent to become a threesome is no longer the same, and there is bound to be a period of adjustment before the new situation is accepted. You may find you feel very dependent, and this need for support will continue for a time after the birth. You will be constantly preoccupied with the baby – will certainly feel very tired, and will possibly be depressed too – so that you may be unable to give your husband the care and attention he needs. You may find you both have unspoken fears about sex; you may not feel desire for a while; he may be frightened of hurting you.

If you both decide before the birth that initially it will be your partner's job to care for you both by taking on as much of the shopping, cooking and cleaning as he can manage, the early weeks will be much easier for all of you, and your relationship with each other will become much more of a partnership and therefore much more serene; whereas, if you desperately try to cope with everything *and* the baby, relations can be strained. Either way, fathers need to be involved from the beginning and communication is the key, so try and talk it through.

The older child

Another relationship which may change following the birth of a new baby is the one you have with your older children. Many parents worry and feel guilty before the birth of a second baby, particularly if there is a small age gap between the two children. They feel that perhaps they are being unfair to their firstborn, displacing him whilst he is still a baby.

Toddlers may show their jealousy by reverting to babyish habits – waking at night and forgetting their toilet training. They may not show their animosity to the baby directly, but will become 'difficult' in their attempts to capture *your* interest. Even if there is a gap of many years, older children can show their anxiety and fear of being displaced in your affection by becoming truculent and untidy. It is difficult for firstborn children to appreciate that all children in a family are loved, and only time, plus your continued reassurance, will show them that they mean as much to you as their rival. Of course life has to continue, and chores have to be done – but many early relationship problems can happily be dealt with by touching and cuddling and *showing* each other that although the pattern of interaction has changed, affection and love are still there.

Preventing loneliness

Loneliness may be something you never experienced before your first baby was born. It is not until you are actually home – alone with your baby – that you might suddenly feel very isolated and miss adult conversation and company.

To avoid this, it is a good idea to exchange telephone numbers with some of the other expectant mothers in your antenatal class, so that even if you are the first among your own friends or family to have a baby you will still be able to communicate with someone who appreciates how difficult those early weeks can be. The telephone can be a lifeline, even though it is not the same as human company.

Ask your health visitor or doctor if they know of someone who has recently had a baby and who lives nearby; start conversations with other mothers when you visit the local baby clinic, and ask if they have a 'Mother and Baby Club'. Find out if the local National Child Birth Trust has a postnatal support group in your area or perhaps the National Housewives Register has a group meeting in your neighbourhood. It might be helpful if you tell yourself that you are not the only new mother who is feeling so alone, and that probably most of the women you see in the shops and in the street with tiny babies are feeling the same way.

Postnatal depression

Most women will pass safely through the postnatal period with nothing more than a mild attack of the blues to bother them. For the remaining 10 per cent or so, a more severe form of emotional upset – postnatal depression – can become a long lasting, trying condition. It does not necessarily begin immediately after the baby is born, indeed it may be several weeks or months before it occurs, but its effect on both mother and family is shattering.

Symptoms of depression

Most postnatally depressed women complain of extreme exhaustion – not just the normal postnatal fatigue but something much more intense and continuous. Sadness and weepiness, a sense of inadequacy, tension and anxiety, irrational fears – these are all symptoms of this very common disorder. Some women complain of physical symptoms too – palpitations, dizziness, aching all over, an inability to sleep in spite of their tiredness, or a complete loss of libido (sexual interest). Sometimes a woman will complain of loss of appetite and will lose weight; yet other women will feel the need to go on frequent eating binges, putting on excessive weight instead of losing it. Women suffering from postnatal depression are often unsmiling, very irritable, short tempered and can experience terrifying moments when they really hate their children and desperately want to hurt them.

Feelings of aggression

You may have thought that your baby would sleep for 20 hours each day, only waking every so often for a feed, so that you would have plenty of time for yourself. It is quite a shock to realize that even a two-week-old baby wants a social life and can stay awake for hours on end needing constant entertainment, driving you, meanwhile, to distraction. All normal parents will admit to terrifying moments when their baby pushes them to the brink of violence. Thankfully most of us step back from this, horrified by our feelings. Try not to feel too guilty about them; instead learn to recognize the signs, counter them with the crisis relaxation techniques given later on page 42 and find someone sympathetic in whom you can confide.

Dealing with depression

It is useless to tell a depressed woman to 'pull herself together' – she cannot do it. At a time when she feels she should be glowing with happiness and contentment, enjoying her new baby and family and coping with all the domestic chores as efficiently and easily as before her pregnancy, she finds herself in a slough of despondency and hopelessness.

Fortunately postnatal depression is now recognized much more frequently by doctors and health visitors – and by mothers and their families too. It can be treated and women can be helped over this distressing period. Psychotherapy, anti-depressant pills and hormone treatment are all used with good results. If you are still breastfeeding, your doctor will take this into account and only prescribe treatment which is safe for the baby. Talking to people about your feelings can help enormously – your health visitor, other women in the clinic, friends with older children – they will all understand and will help you realize that emotional illness can be a part of childbirth for some people, and, for the vast majority of them, can be dealt with swiftly.

Getting back to normal

The passing of time soon brings its compensations. The early weeks of constant caring gradually change when you see that first dazzling smile, when your baby 'talks' back to you, and follows your movements around the room. Suddenly your baby is beginning to learn to socialize and you realize that normal life goes on outside the confines of parenthood, and there will be moments which you will treasure and which will remain with you even when your 'baby' has begun to earn his own living!

At the end of the first three months the continuous hard physical work of caring for a new baby begins to be worth it – and both you and your partner will be glad to be parents after all.

THE IMPORTANCE
OF RELAXATION

During pregnancy your preparation for labour may have included learning relaxation techniques which help the body to cope with stress and work more efficiently. Even if you produce a large family, the total number of hours spent in labour during a lifetime is tiny, but the lessons learned in your antenatal classes can be readily applied to your life in general, and especially to those early days and weeks following birth.

Babies are born knowing instinctively how to relax; you will feel your own baby's deep relaxation when you hold him or her close to your body. You know how to relax too; every night when you drift into sleep the muscles of your body stop working and relax. Even without sleep you know how to relax: when you lie on the beach or in your back garden, soaking up the summer sun, your body comfortably supported, your muscles have no need to work and they relax. Faced with a stressful situation, however, you become tense – and your body will always react in the same way, regardless of the cause. Even babies respond to stress – pain, discomfort, loneliness, the fear of being dropped, or anger at not being fed.

The effects of stress

The stresses and strains we experience as we pass through childhood and adolescence to reach adult life produce muscle tensions which can give rise to postural distortions; raised tense shoulders, clenched fists, jaws clamped tightly together, pressed lips, furrowed forehead, and altered respiration. Mental turmoil often leads to physical tension and the vicious circle is established: the body reacts to the anxieties felt within by hunching, clenching, tightening, and gritting; this leads to aches and pains and more emotional distress. This reaction to stress is one of your body's primitive reflexes. You sense danger, and at once your muscles tense, ready to fight or run away. Other responses include sweating, pallor, pounding heart, dry mouth and faster, deeper respiration.

During pregnancy, the prospect of labour and delivery stand

before you rather like the highest mountain of a range; once you have climbed it and reached its peak (the moment of birth) you imagine that the descent to new parenthood will be easy. As we have seen, you may in fact be totally unprepared for the reality of the early days and weeks of your new baby's life. Tension and fatigue seem to increase hourly; when your baby wakes for the fourth time one night your body reacts by producing the primitive stress response. You try to pacify him with tight, raised shoulders, anxiety and tiredness wrinkling your face – and a coiled spring of tension within you that may make you want to shake the wretched child back to sleep.

Reciprocal relaxation

Fortunately there is a very useful law of the body called reciprocal relaxation which can help you move away from the tense, hunched posture invoked by stress. While one group of muscles works to perform a movement, the opposite group has to relax. This is a physiological fact that you can use to help yourself. For example, to bring ease and comfort to tightly clenched teeth, you can work the muscles which oppose the upward pull on your jaw. Try this: Clench your teeth. Then, with your lips just together, drag the lower jaw down – stop doing it and then notice the new position of your teeth, slightly apart. Your jaws are now relaxed.

The Mitchell Method of Physiological Relaxation

Picture your reaction to the extreme stress of fear. Your shoulders are up, arms pulled into your sides, elbows bent and hands clenched, legs ready to run, body crouched forward, chin tucked into your chest, your face distorted. The following sequence of movements – a technique known as 'physiological relaxation' – is the direct opposite to those your body makes to achieve the tension posture. Because of the law of reciprocal relaxation, following each individual movement, tense parts of your body will *always* become relaxed. Bit by bit you can take your body away from the posture of tension to the position of ease and relaxation.

Lie down comfortably on your back with your head and thighs supported by pillows.

1 Shoulders Pull your shoulders towards your feet – then stop pulling. Register the new position of ease in your mind – your shoulders are relaxed.

2 Arms Push your elbows out and open – stop pushing when you feel your position to be comfortable; register this position – your arms are relaxed.

3 Hands Let them rest comfortably on your thighs or tummy. Stretch the fingers so that they are long and straight; stop. Notice their new position – loosely curled and relaxed.

4 Hips Tighten your buttocks and press your knees out sideways. Stop doing it – notice the relaxed sensation in your hips.

5 Knees Lift your heels; stop doing it – and register the comfortable feeling in your knees and thighs.

6 Feet Press your feet away from your face. Stop doing it – and notice comfortable feet dangling on the ends of your legs.

7 Body Press your body into the support behind you; stop doing it – and register the pleasant sensation of relaxation in your abdomen.

8 Head Press your head into the support behind it – stop pressing – and notice how this movement has relaxed your neck and upper shoulders. (If you want to try this while sitting in a chair and your head is not supported, let it tilt forward slightly till it reaches a comfortable position.)

9 Face (a) your jaw: drag you lower jaw down; stop doing it – then notice the pleasant feeling of comfort that you have when your upper and lower sets of teeth are resting slightly apart.

(b) your mouth: stretch your lips sideways in a little smile, pout your lips forwards very quickly and then notice the pleasing sensation of soft warm lips just lightly touching each other.

(c) your eyes: your lids are resting comfortably over your eyes. You may even want to close them.

(d) your forehead: imagine that someone is stroking it and smoothing away the lines of tension.

Relaxing your jaw
Clenched teeth (right) often accompany tension. Drag your jaw down keeping your lips touching (centre); then stop and let your teeth rest slightly apart (far right).

Breathing for relaxation

Because the way you breathe is affected by stress, altering your respiration is one of the easiest ways of inducing relaxation. You tend to breathe out as you relax: imagine your reaction to finding a purse that you'd thought you'd lost – with next week's food money in it – you sigh with relief and relax. If you use this response to deal with the many problems which crop up continuously during parenthood, they can often be resolved painlessly. Breathe out and relax at the beginning of a feed if you feel the needle-like pain from a sore nipple. Breathe out and relax when you realize that you have run out of disposable nappies. Breathe out and relax when your toddler unravels a completely new toilet roll or empties the contents of his pot on the floor.

Use your breathing to increase the depth of your relaxation. Make it slow, calm and quiet. Concentrate on the outward breath – empty your chest – pause – and then let only as much air into your lungs as you need at that particular moment – do not force more and more air into your chest.

The beauty of the Mitchell Method is that it always works, day or night, whatever your position and whatever you are doing, (washing, feeding the baby, waiting for a bus). It is not always necessary to lie down in a darkened room surrounded by silence to be able to relax. You can take your hunched shoulders away from their tense position by simply moving them in the opposite direction. (See Further Reading: **Relaxation**)

Using the Mitchell Method

It is not necessary to run through all the movements every time. Your shoulders, arms, hands and face are usually the first parts of your body to respond to stress – recognise the tension in them and release it by adjusting the stress-induced posture.

Whenever your baby is sleeping, experiment with several comfortable positions to use to rest, doze or sleep yourself. Feeding time gives you a wonderful opportunity to practise relaxation, for tension is catching; if you start nursing your baby while sitting uncomfortably, your back will begin to ache, you may be scared to move in case your baby stops sucking, you will become tense and long for the feed to finish. In turn, your baby may sense this and will become disturbed and restless. Anxiety at the beginning of a feed can delay the 'let down' reflex which makes the milk-producing glands release the milk in your breasts. Use your relaxation to overcome this. Always make sure you are comfortable, close your eyes (if it helps) and consciously run through the body movements to give you total relaxation.

Many mothers find it hard to get back to sleep once they have been disturbed by their baby at night; use your relaxation technique and slow calm breathing to help you float into sleep again. Relaxation is a valuable tool, always there for you to use during crises. Remember, by practising this useful technique, you will be *using* time and not wasting it, and it will become a lifelong legacy of childbirth.

Crisis measures

For those difficult moments when you reach breaking point, try this emergency relaxation measure.

Breathe out – then, breathing naturally:

Face Smooth away worry lines – teeth apart.

Shoulders Down – stop – feel it.

Hands Long stretched fingers – stop – feel it.

Relaxing feeding positions

Left: Sit cross-legged on the floor with your back supported against a wall. Raise your baby by placing a pillow across your knees.

Above: Lie on your side with your baby against you. Support your head and shoulders with two pillows and place one between your knees.

Comfortable relaxation positions

1 Lie on your front with a pillow under your hips. This position is particularly useful for the immediate postnatal period when you may have uncomfortable perineal stitches or haemorrhoids.

2 Lie flat on your back with legs apart and palms upwards. Support your head with a pillow and place another under your thighs.

3 An alternative to the above position is to raise your legs by resting your feet on a low stool or coffee table, with one pillow placed under your heels and another under your head.

4 You can relax in the middle of doing the chores for a few minutes by sitting at a table with your knees wide apart and feet flat on the floor, resting your head on your arms.

It is helpful to relax for five to ten minutes after you have completed your daily postnatal exercise sessions. The positions suggested in the Daily Programmes (pages 62, 89 and 112) are only given as guides; you could use whichever position described here seems most comfortable at the time.

EASY RELAXATION EXERCISES

UNCURLING
Stand up and bend forward so that your shoulders and arms hang heavily. Stay there, resting and breathing quietly. Slowly uncurl, bringing your body upwards. When you are straight stand still for a moment, breathing quietly. You may like to arch your back, supporting your waist with your hands. You can also do this exercise sitting in a chair with your knees wide apart.

SHOULDER CIRCLING

(This exercise can be done standing or sitting.) Circle your shoulders backwards, first one, then the other and then both together. Finish with them both down in a relaxed position.

ARM STRETCHING

S-T-R-E-T-C-H your arms as high as you can above your head; then stop and relax. You can do this stretching movement sitting down, standing up or lying on your bed.

GETTING STARTED

EXERCISES
0 TO 6 WEEKS

First thoughts on exercise

Whether you had a long or short, easy or difficult labour, probably the last thing you will feel like doing immediately after your baby is born is to begin your postnatal exercises. Don't worry – you do not need to start a vigorous programme immediately; there are a few simple movements though that will make you feel more comfortable.

Some women may have little or no discomfort, while others will notice heavy legs, a sore throbbing perineum and possibly backache. For those who have had a Caesarean section there may be intense burning pain over and around the line of the incision. Whatever your type of delivery, you will probably notice that every time you try to change your position during the first few hours, there will be a flow of blood (lochia) from the vagina. Because of this you may, mistakenly, feel nervous of moving, let alone beginning your exercises. If you have stitches in your pelvic floor or abdomen, you may also be worried that they will come apart if you move too energetically. However, you can be quite sure that the exercises given in the first part (0-48 hours) of this section are not only safe but essential for your speedy recovery and you can even do the first four while still in the delivery room.

Make the most of your few days away from domestic chores; rest when you can, but try to fit in a few exercises three times a day. As a bare minimum, try to get into the habit of pulling your tummy muscles in and drawing your pelvic floor muscles in and up while you feed your baby. Aim at 20 contractions per feed done in groups of four (see pages 49 and 52). All the exercises in the first section, except for the first two, should be continued at home.

Being careful

Once you feel you are able to start the slightly harder exercises there are a few important rules to observe:
1 Never exercise to the point of pain or exhaustion.
2 Stop if you feel nauseated, dizzy or faint.
3 Learn to listen to your body so that you do not inadvertently strain your weak muscles.
4 Don't exercise last thing at night when you are feeling tired, or if you are ill.

A warning

There are two exercises which should **never** be attempted during this postnatal period. They are:
1 Lying flat on your back with both legs straight on the floor, and then trying to lift them together.
2 Lying flat on your back with both legs straight and attempting to sit up.

Afterpains

Many new mothers experience painful uterine contractions ('afterpains') for the first few days while they are breastfeeding. This is due to the release of the hormone oxytocin, which shrinks the uterus as it stimulates the 'let down' reflex in the breast. Women who are bottle feeding may notice these contractions when they begin abdominal exercises. Although uncomfortable these are normal and beneficial. Use the following exercises to 'breathe your way through' the pain (see page 49).

THE FIRST FORTY-EIGHT HOURS

BREATHING AND FIRST ABDOMINAL EXERCISE

This exercise improves your circulation, gently strengthens your abdominal muscles and helps you to relax.

Lie comfortably on your back with your knees bent, resting your hand on your abdomen. Take a slow deep breath in through your nose, then sigh the air out through your slightly parted lips and draw your abdominal muscles in at the end of the outward breath. Some women are surprised that these muscles should be pulled in at this point, but it is in fact part of the natural breathing pattern. Once you have learnt this sequence, you will then be able to use breathing out to help you relax.

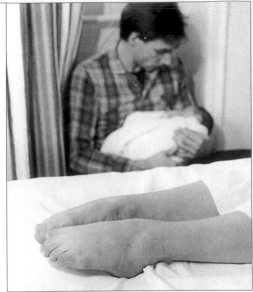

FOOT EXERCISES

These two movements will improve your leg circulation; they are particularly important if you have to stay in bed.

Lie comfortably with your knees straight and together (above). Bend and stretch your feet up and down at the ankles. This should be done briskly and for about 30 seconds at a time.

Move your feet about 30 cm (12 in) apart. Then circle your feet ten times in each direction (right and below).

PELVIC ROCKING

This exercise promotes good posture, firms the abdominal muscles and can help ease backache, constipation, and post-Caesarean section abdominal wind.

Lie comfortably with your knees bent and together. Squeeze your buttocks together tilting them upwards. Blow out, drawing in your abdominal muscles and pressing your back firmly onto the bed. Hold for four counts. When you feel able to, this exercise can be made more difficult by holding the muscle contractions for longer – up to ten counts, and then including the basic pelvic floor exercise (page 52) with your pelvic rocking.

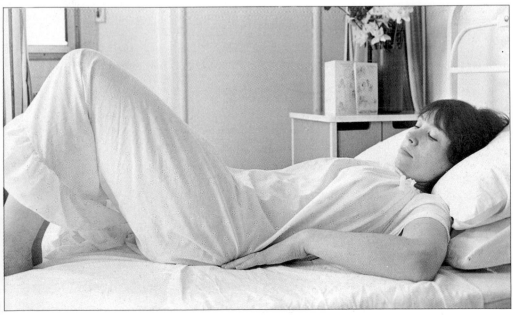

BASIC PELVIC FLOOR EXERCISE

This important exercise strengthens the pelvic floor hammock, and it can help to relieve pain by promoting the absorption of swelling.

Lie with your knees bent and apart. At first you may be unable to feel your vagina, so start by tightening your anal sphincter. Hold this, then let it relax. Later, imagine a tampon is falling out of your vagina. Draw your vaginal muscles in and up as if to grip it, hold, then relax. Now repeat this quick movement more slowly, holding the muscle contraction for four counts. Try to do these contractions a minimum of four times every 15 minutes. In the same way that you have to train yourself to become used to a new body posture – bottom and tummy tucked in, ribs well lifted – so you have to become aware of the position of your pelvic floor – your *internal* posture.

You can test your progress by trying to stop the flow of urine towards the end of your stream. You will gradually regain this control.

TESTING YOUR ABDOMINAL MUSCLES

If you turn back to page 17 you will see that the two sides of your abdominal 'corset' nearly always separate towards the end of your pregnancy to accommodate your growing baby. After your baby's birth this gap can be an indication of the strength of the recti abdominis. You cannot feel the separation properly unless you make your muscles work hard. To test yourself, lie on your back with your knees bent up high – pull your abdominal muscles in, lift your head and shoulders and stretch one arm as far as you can towards your feet. Put the fingers of your other hand just below your umbilicus and feel for the space. Initially almost everyone will have a gap at least two fingers wide – and many people will have a much wider space, three to four fingers wide. As your muscles recover and become stronger, this will gradually close until the gap is so small and tight that you can only insert the tip of one finger.

LEG SLIDING

This is a very efficient tummy toning exercise – it makes both your vertical abdominal muscles (the recti abdominis) work very hard, shortening them and helping to close the gap between them.

Lie comfortably on your back with your knees bent, feet flat and hands behind your head. Pull in your abdominal muscles and tuck your chin on your chest so that the back of your waist is pressed very firmly on to the bed. Keeping your back on the bed, slide both feet away from you as far as you can without allowing your back to arch up. Still keeping your back flat on the bed, slowly draw your feet towards your buttocks again.

Initially you may not be able to slide your feet more than a few inches without your back arching, which demonstrates how weak your abdominal muscles are. Gradually your control will improve so that eventually you should be able to straighten and bend your legs completely without losing your back control. Start by doing this exercise four times and gradually increase to twelve.

CURL-UPS

This movement strengthens your vertical abdominal muscles.

Lie on your back with your knees bent up high. Blow out and tilt your pelvis up by pulling in your abdominal muscles and drawing your buttocks together while tucking your chin on your chest. Lift your head and shoulders as high as you can, stretching your hands towards your feet. Hold this position for four counts – and then lower slowly. Start with six and increase to twelve.

A USEFUL RESTING POSITION AND BUTTOCK TONER

Many women do not realize that once again they can lie flat on their fronts. To do this really comfortably you will need to use two pillows – one under your waist and the other under your head and shoulders, making a space for your breasts. Of course, this position does not flatten or strengthen your abdomen in any way, but it is said to help the uterus to return to its normal position over the bladder. If you have a tender episiotomy, haemorrhoids or backache, you will find that rhythmical buttock squeezing while lying on your front may help relieve your discomfort. Everyone will eventually find this a wonderfully restful position, even those who have had a Caesarean section. It will allow you to relax fully without uncomfortable pressure and could begin toning up flabby buttocks.

THE POST-CAESAREAN MOTHER

There are two kinds of Caesarean birth:

Elective – you knew in advance that you would have to have a Caesarean section for your baby to be born safely.

Emergency – the decision to help your baby out by Caesarean section was only taken during labour.

You may have had a general anaesthetic for the operation and could be a bit 'chesty' afterwards because of its effect on your lungs. Alternatively you may have had an epidural anaesthetic and will have been awake as your baby was born. No matter why or how you had a Caesarean section, you will feel very sore around the site of the operation and will find it very difficult to move easily because of the pain. You are going to need much more help during the first few days.

Special Post-operative Exercises

You will feel much better if you do these simple exercises as soon as possible. They will improve your circulation and are relaxing. Lie comfortably on your back, well supported by pillows, with your legs straight.

1 Bend and stretch your ankles vigorously 30 times.

2 Circle your ankles (10 times in each direction).

3 Press your knees down hard on to the bed and relax (10 times).

4 Draw your buttocks tightly together and relax (10 times).

5 Bend and stretch your knees alternately (10 times).

6 Practise deep breathing, filling and emptying both lungs completely. Try a 'huffing' breath outwards, while supporting your incision with both hands, if you need to clear your throat.

7 If you are 'chesty', you will need to cough properly. Probably the most comfortable position for coughing is sitting with your legs over the side of your bed or on a high chair. Separate your knees, support your wound with a pillow, *lean forwards* and cough with a sharp 'huff'.

A pillow placed under your thighs will prevent you from slipping down the bed and another resting across your wound will help prevent too much pain as you feed your baby as shown, or you may like to tuck your baby under your arm with his feet behind you.

Hints for comfort

If you have had a Caesarean section your needs are somewhat different from those of mothers who have had normal deliveries, and you will probably receive plenty of help from the nursing staff during your first few days.

Feeding your baby

You may find that your most comfortable position is in bed, well-propped up with pillows, or sitting comfortably in an armchair.

Getting in and out of bed

Make sure that your bed is as low as possible or use a stool. To get out of bed, shuffle your bottom to the edge of the bed and lift your legs one at a time over the side (using your hands if needed). Separate your knees, support your wound with your hands, lean forwards and slowly stand up. The first few times you will need some help. After a few days you will be able to lie flat. Then it is easiest to roll on your side to get out of bed – bend your knees and use your arms to push yourself up before swinging your legs over the edge and standing up.

To get back into bed, lower your bottom on to the mattress *right next to your pillows*. Make sure you are well on to the bed and not on the edge. Now lift your legs one at a time on to the bed, using your hands if necessary.

Standing and walking

You will probably have to support your wound with your hands in the beginning – but if you can straighten up it is usually less painful. Practise deep slow breathing as you move around the room and go to the lavatory – this breathing is relaxing and can help relieve the pain.

Pain

After your Caesarean section you will probably have pain from at least three sources: your wound, 'afterpains' (see page 48) and abdominal wind.

Solutions

1 You will certainly be offered pain-killers. Don't reject these if you need them – there is no virtue in suffering unnecessarily.
2 Gently stroke your tummy using your right hand to move upwards from your right groin to your waist, across your waist towards your left side, and down to your left groin. Repeat this movement, which pushes the wind along your large bowel, until you are able to pass it.
3 Pelvic rocking (see page 51) will also ease wind discomfort.

Normal postnatal exercising

Your obstetric physiotherapist will guide you. You will probably only be a few days behind the other mothers, but because you have had a major operation as well as having had a baby it will take you longer to recover from the birth than your friends who have had vaginal deliveries. It is important to accept that you will need to take things easy for the first four weeks or longer.

At home

When you first go home, rest as much as possible and try to make the household chores wait until you feel more fit. If friends offer to shop, clean or cook for you, or take your other children off your hands for a while, do accept their help.

As the weeks go by you will find that you gradually feel stronger and more able to cope – you will have caught up with mothers whose babies were born normally.

AT HOME

BACK AND BUTTOCK TONER

This exercise not only firms your buttocks but also encourages the small but important muscles of your lower back to work.

Lie flat on your front on the floor with your head resting on your hands. (If your breasts are tender use two pillows, one under your head and the other under your waist.) Keeping your knees straight, lift your left leg without allowing your pelvis to twist backwards. Hold for four counts and then lower slowly. Repeat with the right leg. Do this six times with each leg, increasing to twelve. If you experience back pain whilst doing this exercise put a further one or two pillows under your waist.

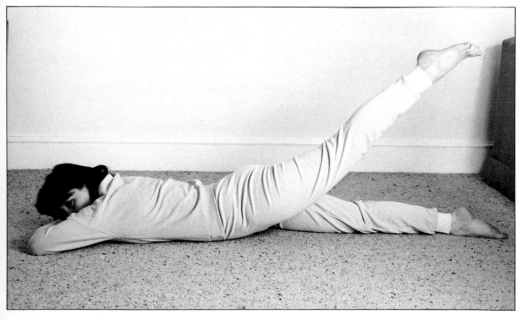

QUICK RELAXATION AND BACK MOBILIZER

This useful exercise can be done almost anywhere and at any time to achieve quick relaxation. It has the added benefit of loosening your tired, tense back muscles.

Sit straight on a chair or stool with your knees and feet wide apart. Curl forward, breathing out so that your arms and head are hanging heavily down. Relax there for a few moments, breathing quietly, feeling the tension draining out of you. Then slowly uncurl your body, straightening your lower back and waist first, followed by your shoulders and finally your head. Hold this relaxed but upright position for a moment, making sure that your shoulders are not hunched up by your ears. Repeat this a few times until your back feels comfortable and easy.

WAIST WHITTLER

With this exercise, you are working the muscles at the sides and front of your waist.

Sit up straight on a chair with your knees and feet apart. Hold your abdomen in firmly and keep your bottom on the chair. Bend sideways to the right, stretching your hand towards the floor. Keeping your tummy flat, straighten up slowly, then relax your abdomen. Repeat the movement to the left.

Be very careful not to allow your body to move forwards or back; the movement should be restricted to a sideways bend, as if your body is fixed between two walls, front and back. Do this four times to each side, increasing to twelve.

PECTORAL TONER

When you first do this exercise it will probably be helpful to watch yourself in a mirror. You should see a brisk movement of the muscles underlying the breast, and some women may notice their breasts move too.

Sit up straight on a chair with your knees and feet apart and your arms lifted and bent in front of you; hold your upper arms with the opposite hand. Now push the palms of your hands firmly against your upper arms and stop. You will feel your pectoral muscles contracting sharply and then relaxing.

WAIST TWISTER

This exercise uses the diagonal (oblique) muscles of the abdominal corset, firming your tummy and helping to pull in your waist.

Sitting in the same position as for the Pectoral Toner on the previous page, hold your abdomen in hard. Keeping your bottom fixed on the chair and your back erect, twist your body round to the right as far as you can; hold for four counts, then swing round to the left; come back to your starting position and relax your abdominal muscles. Do this six times to each side increasing to twelve.

DAILY PROGRAMME

These sections are designed to help you see at a glance which exercises to do and how many times to do them. Unless otherwise stated, do these sets of exercises *twice a day*. Asterisks mark the most important ones, so when you have very little time you should at least try to fit these in.

The first 48 hours

BREATHING AND FIRST ABDOMINAL EXERCISE
Circulation, abdominal muscles, relaxation
page 49
Do this 4 times every so often

FOOT EXERCISES
Leg circulation page 50
Do the first exercise for 30 seconds, and the second exercise 20 times in each direction, 3 to 4 times a day

The first 48 hours and at home

* PELVIC ROCKING
Abdominal and buttock muscles
page 51
6 to 10 rocks, 3 to 4 times a day in hospital, twice a day at home

* BASIC PELVIC FLOOR EXERCISE
Pelvic floor muscles
page 52
4 times every hour

* LEG SLIDING
Vertical abdominal muscles
page 53
4 to 12 times, 3 to 4 times a day in hospital, and twice a day at home

* CURL-UPS
Vertical abdominal muscles
page 54
6 to 12 times, 3 to 4 times a day in hospital, and twice a day at home

RESTING POSITION AND BUTTOCK TONER
Buttocks, backache page 54
Use the resting position for 15 to 30 minutes.
Squeeze your buttocks 10 times every so often during this rest.

TESTING YOUR ABDOMINAL MUSCLES
page 52
Try doing this test once or twice a week and note the gradual change

POST-CAESAREAN MOTHERS
Remember to do your additional exercises on page 56

At home only

BACK AND BUTTOCK TONER
Buttocks and lower back
page 57
6 to 12 times (each leg)

QUICK RELAXATION AND BACK MOBILIZER
Quick relaxation and backache page 58
Do several times

WAIST WHITTLER
Side and front waist muscles
page 59
4 to 12 times each side

PECTORAL TONER
Pectoral muscles page 60
10 times

WAIST TWISTER
Oblique abdominal muscles page 61
6 to 12 times each side

Post work-out relaxation

Leaning forward on to a table, resting your head on your hands (see page 43). Practise your simple relaxation technique (see page 40). Rest like this for as long as possible.

YOUR BABY'S PHYSICAL NEEDS

Having left the enfolding security of the womb for the strange, noisy and vast space of the outside world, your baby will need your warmth and reassurance to help her to adjust to her new environment. Sudden careless movements will startle her and cause her to throw out her arms involuntarily in panic. Babies like calm, confident handling; being wrapped and held securely nearly always soothes and relaxes them. Swaddling is a time-honoured way of making a very new baby feel warm and contented – but should be avoided if your baby has an unstable 'clicky' hip.

Points to consider

In the first six weeks, babies' material needs are few – food, adequate warmth and clothing, and somewhere comfortable to sleep. It is worthwhile remembering this, for you will probably feel rather daunted when you walk into your nearest baby shop and see all the paraphernalia that manufacturers seem to believe essential for your child's normal development.

You will probably already have some ideas as to the choice of bed and transport for your baby, based on considerations such as whether you have a car, are going back to work and will be leaving your baby with others, have older children, like to stay at home, like to walk everywhere, are glad to make do with hand-me-downs or want to have only the newest and best.

You may have taken advice on the safest and best-designed equipment and toys, but there are some important points to consider from your own physical point of view and also for the development of your baby, which you will not be able to learn from the catalogues.

Keeping your baby amused

It is now recognized that a full term newborn baby can see and follow movement with her eyes; she can hear, taste and smell, and within a matter of days has learnt to identify the face, voice and smell of her mother. She is, however, completely dependent, and it is only by crying that she is able to convey her needs. Her movements are jerky, uncontrolled and often governed by infant reflexes. She is a passive observer, learning through her senses about the world around her.

By about three or four weeks of age she starts to watch her mother and father intently, following them with her eyes, and her own face becomes increasingly alert. She is interested in movement, particularly that of a face, and turns her head towards light, and sometimes to a nearby sound, such as music or a voice. Her body and limbs still remain generally curled up and her hands can only open involuntarily. But by the time she is six weeks old she will enjoy searching her mother's and father's faces – especially their eyes and mouths – and will often hold their gaze for several moments, perhaps even breaking into a lopsided smile.

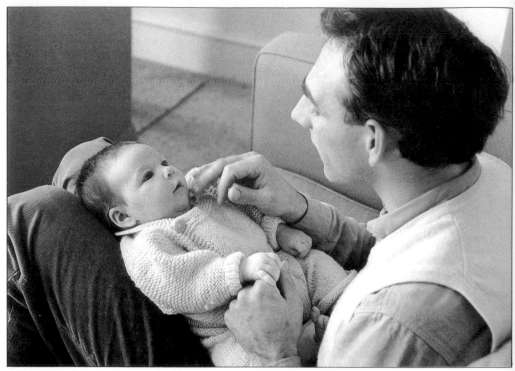

Looking and listening

At this stage a baby does not need toys to play with – she is totally absorbed in learning about her environment, especially the people most important to her. Of course you can't always be available to her if she lies awake, so you can try taping some large photographs to the side of her bed or a frieze on the wall nearest where she spends most of her day. A mobile, balloons or a soft toy suspended securely about 20 cm (8 in) above her bed may provide movement and colour to catch her interest and help develop her sensory awareness. A music box playing a soothing tune helps to settle some babies. Remember, however, that you are by far the most exciting thing in your baby's world.

Carrying your baby

Slings (or harnesses) are a comforting and natural way to carry babies. They enjoy the warmth, the reassuring sound of a heart-beat and the motion. Being carried in this way is also physically good for them, as it encourages head control and a healthy position of the hips. In Nigeria, where this is the most common way of transporting babies, congenital dislocation of the hips is hardly ever seen. Slings are obviously ideal for crowded shops with escalators or walks which are muddy, bumpy or stepped. They are often an answer for the unsettled or colicky baby, who may cease crying and even fall asleep while her mother manages a few chores.

Choosing a sling

If you decide to buy a sling, make sure it has shoulder straps which are well padded and adjustable. If you are short and your partner tall, when either of you wears it you will each need to

Left: A baby has begun to focus by six to eight weeks. Remember that your face is your baby's most exciting plaything at this age.

adjust the supporting straps so that your baby's head is as near to your respective chins as is comfortable. This will minimize strain to your backs. Make sure it is not worn to the side, as prolonged carrying of a weight on one side is almost bound to cause backache particularly at this stage.

In their first weeks, babies' heads need some support but this will diminish after three or four months and will no longer be necessary by six months, so choose a sling that can be adjusted accordingly. One of the best slings has an adjustable inner pouch for the young baby, and an outer pouch for the bigger baby or toddler. A newborn baby nestles in the inner pouch and is almost completely enfolded by the outer one, which acts as head support and extra warmth for the body and limbs. The straps adjust and are well padded, so that it can be used just as successfully to carry a tired toddler on the back as a new baby on the front. The alternatives, which are often cheaper, are sometimes only useful for a brief period while the baby is small – the head support is often no more than an inadequate piece of padding added on to the back support, and the design is often unsuitable to take the weight of a heavier baby with comfort.

If your baby dislikes the sling

Very occasionally there are babies who do not enjoy slings and protest as soon as they are put in them. There is also the

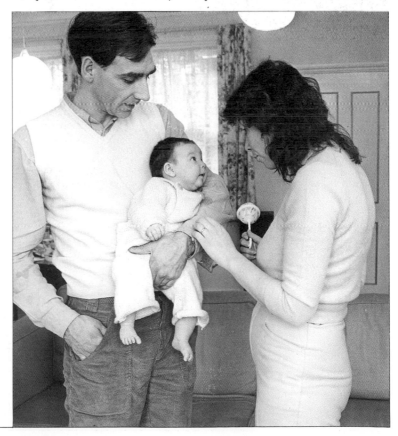

Try this secure way of holding your small baby. It will leave you with a free hand while allowing your baby to watch her surroundings as you move about.

odd baby who will not tolerate long spells in one and demands to be taken out and allowed to move before being put in again. You will soon learn what she likes or dislikes, and obviously it is not worth persevering too long once you have established the sling to be the cause of her displeasure. If you can possibly try your baby in the sling of your choice before buying, then it is worth doing so. Most large stores will actually encourage you to do this.

Carrying with one arm

There is another excellent way of carrying your baby without a sling, but which still leaves one arm free. Using your preferred hand, place your forearm down the front of your baby's trunk with her head resting into the crook of your elbow. Her underside arm must be behind your forearm for safety, and your hand can then hold her between the legs. This position stimulates your baby's head control and vision, and you may also find it is an excellent position for bringing up a burp (see page 65).

Winding your baby

Wind is often mistakenly given as the reason for your baby's crying. While all babies, particularly very young ones, do swallow air as they feed (especially if they are bottlefed), and certainly swallow air if they are left to cry, it is unlikely to be the cause of any incessant crying. Much more likely reasons are

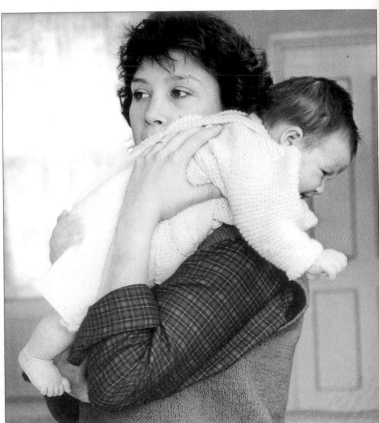

You can soothe or 'wind' your baby by holding her over your shoulder so her trunk is elongated, then gently rub her back with your free hand.

Positions for
winding

hunger, feelings of loneliness or overstimulation, feeling hot or cold, fear of loud noises or being dropped, and dislike of being undressed.

However, if you are in doubt about the reason for your baby's crying after you have fed, changed and cuddled her, it is possible that air trapped in her stomach may be causing her discomfort. Put her over your shoulder and very gently pat or rub her back, making sure that you drape her well over the top of your shoulder with her arms hanging down your back. By doing this you are lengthening her trunk so that the wind can escape more readily. If your baby likes to spend a lot of time like this, it is a good idea to try to alternate shoulders, so that you don't get a stiff aching neck on one side.

Another traditional winding position is to hold your baby

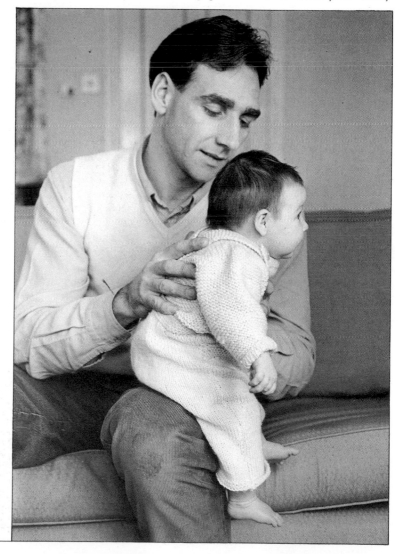

Even if your baby is breastfed, her father can help by taking over at the end of the feed to wind and change her.

67

with one hand open across her chest, supporting her head at the chin with your wide open thumb and index finger. Lean your baby slightly forward from the hips while straightening and lengthening her trunk with the supporting hand. At the same time gently rub or pat her back. As your baby may bring back a mouthful of food with the bubble of wind, it is a good idea to protect your clothes with a nappy or towel.

Do not continue trying to extract a burp from your baby for too long – five minutes is plenty. Any wind that is going to escape from the stomach will do so in this time, so if she continues to cry, try to think of the other possible reasons for her unhappiness.

'Three-month colic'   If you find that your baby is fretful and tense over a period

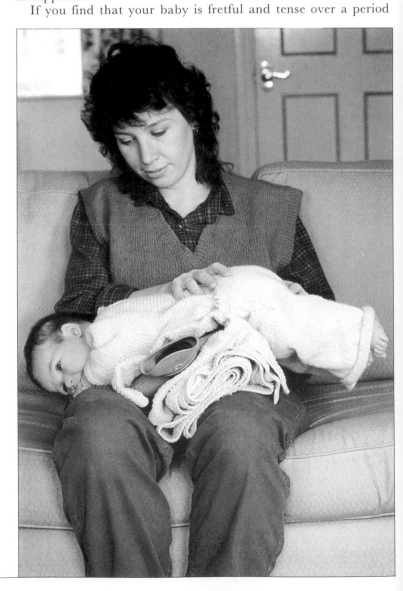

A restless baby can often be soothed in this position. The warmth of a wrapped hot water bottle under her tummy and the comfort of a hand on her back will often send her to sleep at last.

of a few days at a regular time, particularly the evening, and that in spite of running through all the possible causes of discomfort she is still difficult to pacify for more than a few minutes, you may suspect that colic is the cause. Parents find this distressing problem very wearing, but babies generally grow out of this phase by about three months. Discuss it with your health visitor or doctor; in the meantime many parents find that using the following method can soothe a restless baby quite successfully: fill a rubber hot water bottle and wrap it in a soft towel or nappy. Test that it is not uncomfortably hot – babies can be burned so easily. Lay this lengthwise across your lap and then lay your baby on her front over it, with the warmth under her tummy. She will probably like to be gently rocked or stroked at the same time.

Baby massage

Most of us enjoy the soothing effect of gentle massage, and babies seem to be no exception. Choose a time when she is warm, comfortable and well fed. A little talcum powder or pure oil on her skin will help your hand movements, which should be smooth and slow with gentle pressure. Stroking downwards along the length of her abdomen or back will give both of you pleasure. She will probably also enjoy downward stroking along her arms and legs. This baby massage, long used in the East, is thought to enhance a baby's feeling of well-being and increase early parent-child contact.

Sleeping in comfort

A small baby can sleep anywhere that is clean, soft but firm, and draught free but well-ventilated. A smooth box would do just as well as a fancy cot or pram. However if you want to be able to move your baby from room to room as she sleeps, or want to take her out in the car, you will need a bed that is portable. As your back is very vulnerable at this point, weight and size should be considered when you make your choice; both a 'Moses' basket or a mainly-fabric baby nest are light and very easy to manage, but as they are not rigid they cannot be safely fastened into a car. If you want a carrycot so that your baby can go in the back of the car, remember that you will be having to lift it on to the seat for the next five to six months. Try and choose a light one that fits in easily without needing any risky twisting movements of your spine and make sure your baby's head is always carried nearest you as you lift the carrycot. Once on the seat it should be secured in place by restrainer straps (part of which may be able to be used to secure a car seat at a later stage). There are also rearward-facing front or back seats which are held in place by an adult seat belt. These provide extra support for a baby in case of a crash; they are also light, adaptable, easy to transport and comfortable even for the very young baby.

Prams

Most mothers find a pram indispensable in the first few months, and some will continue to use it for several years. For many babies it is their first bed; by gently rocking the pram or taking them out for a walk in it, their parents find they are

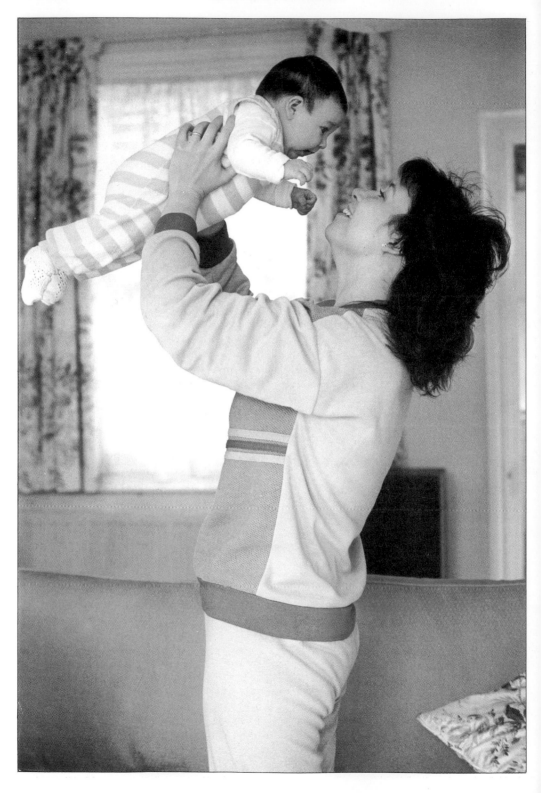

guaranteed almost certain peace. Parents who also have a young toddler can harness the older child to a special pram seat, while piling the shopping into the basket underneath. This way the baby is lulled to sleep, the toddler is taken for an outing, and parents bring home all their shopping with no strain to their backs. Of course, the children cannot be left unattended, even for a moment, since the extra weight of a lively toddler can cause even the sturdiest pram to tilt.

Prams come in a huge range of sizes, just as they vary from the basic to luxurious. Some separate into travel cots and transporters, and still others fold down into buggies. Only you can decide how much and for how long you plan to use a pram, and can evaluate the importance to you of all the accessories available. Remember that the handle should be at a comfortable height when you push it; also, while having the benefit of accommodating an older sleeping baby, a very large carrycot may then be too heavy for you to lift if you need to. Thus your choice of pram should be based upon consideration not only of your baby and your budget but also of your own needs and limitations.

Mother and baby medical examinations

Six weeks will be an important milestone for both you and your baby. Your uterus should by now have returned to its pre-pregnancy shape and size, you will probably notice that you have better control of your abdominal muscles, and the acute pain from your stitches will have faded. Your baby should by this time be rewarding you with wonderful smiles, have established a fairly regular feeding pattern and have better control of her head. It is for all these reasons that six weeks is generally chosen as the ideal time for a doctor to check both of you.

Your postnatal check

You may be seen either at your hospital or by your family doctor. A blood test may be carried out to see if you are anaemic, and your blood pressure will be taken. Your doctor will want to check that your uterus has fully involuted and he will give you a vaginal examination; he may also want to examine your breasts, whether you are breastfeeding or not, and take a cervical smear for testing if you have not had one within the last year. Now is the time to tell him about any of your postnatal problems, especially if you are finding that intercourse is painful, and to ask his advice. He will ask what you have decided to do about contraception and should discuss this with you.

Your baby's six week development check

You will probably have visited your clinic before this, but at six weeks the doctor will give your baby a thorough examination to check her progress. He will record her weight and measure her length and her head and chest circumference. He will look at her eye movements, check her response to sound, and ask you if she has begun to smile. He will also examine her hips and genitals, feel her abdomen and listen to her heart. He will probably check her head control when she is pulled up to sitting. Don't be afraid to mention anything about your baby that is worrying you, however insignificant it may seem.

MAKING PROGRESS

EXERCISES
6 WEEKS TO
3 MONTHS

By this time your baby may have have established the beginnings of a routine and will not be so dependent on you for contact if he wakes between feeds. You will probably have adjusted to the pattern of broken nights and the additional chores and will be able to devote more time and energy to your postnatal recovery.

Your muscles, by no means fully recovered, will have regained some of their strength and you should be ready to move on to stronger, more difficult exercises. In fact, some women will feel ready to tackle this section well before six weeks are up – and there is no reason to hold back if you find that you can cope without undue fatigue or aches and pains. Usually though, and especially if it is your first baby, it does take quite a while to become used to an entirely different life style, and exercises often have to take second or third place on your list of priorities!

Continue using feed times to tone and strengthen your abdominal and pelvic floor muscles. Make sure that you tighten and relax the muscles of the perineum at least twenty times per feed – still in groups of four – holding some contractions for four counts and some just briefly before you relax. Also spend a few moments on your abdominal muscles, holding them in for eight to ten counts while continuing to breathe naturally.

You should now try to set aside a short period of time twice a day to concentrate on stronger ways of working these groups of muscles, while adding new exercises for your back, buttocks and legs, plus your chest and arm muscles.

You will probably find by now that your baby is beginning to respond to being moved and handled. He is becoming less passive and will enjoy simple games and activities to help stimulate his development. As he is now more alert and has some head control you can safely put him in a bouncing cradle, lie him near you as you exercise, or even let him join in.

Your ligaments are now a little stronger and firmer but have by no means recovered fully. You must still take care when bending, twisting and lifting since they can still be easily damaged despite the fact that you may be feeling less exhausted and much more able to cope.

LYING ON THE FLOOR

PELVIC FLOOR AND TUMMY TRIMMER
This exercise will help firm your abdomen and bottom and will also strengthen your pelvic floor.

Lie on the floor with your knees bent; if your baby is awake he can sit on your tummy. Draw your pelvic floor muscles inwards and upwards, concentrating on your vagina. Contract your buttocks so that your bottom lifts up off the floor; blow out, pulling in your abdomen and lifting your head so that your baby can see your face and you can talk to him. Hold this position for four counts, then lower slowly, relaxing all the working muscles. Start with six lifts then progress to twenty. You can also increase the length of time from four to ten counts.

If you still find it difficult to *feel* your pelvic floor working by this stage, it may be helpful after a bath or shower to insert two fingers a couple of inches into your vagina whilst you stand with one foot on the edge of the bath. Now tighten your pelvic floor muscles. You should feel them gripping your fingers. Constant practice will improve your sensation and power.

THE "UP-CURLER"

This very strong exercise will strengthen your straight abdominal muscles and help to draw them closer together.

Lie on your back with your knees bent up high. Tilt your pelvis up by pulling in your abdominal muscles and drawing your buttocks together at the same time. Tuck your chin in, blow out and slowly curl your head and shoulders up off the floor, reaching your arms forward to touch your knees. Hold this position for four counts and then lower yourself slowly back to the floor. Do this six times and increase to twenty.

You can increase the length of time you hold the curled-up position from four counts to 30 seconds, and if you cross your arms over your chest when you do your lift, the exercise will be made even more challenging.

HIP AND WAIST TRIMMER

This exercise uses your oblique abdominal and lower back muscles to slim your waist.

Lie on the floor with your arms away from your sides and your knees bent up high and feet flat. Pull in your abdominal muscles, then take your knees to the left, until your thigh touches the floor. Keep your knees tightly together and your abdomen firmly in, take your knees to the right and then back to the middle; pause, then repeat. It is important to keep both shoulders flat on the floor as you roll your legs from side to side and *very* important to remember to hold in your abdominal muscles throughout the exercise.

Start with six and increase to twenty, progressing the exercise by omitting the pause and increasing the speed of the movement. You may find it helpful to put your hands under your head when you speed up this exercise.

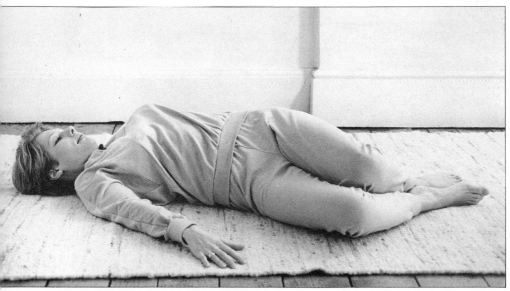

TUMMY FLATTENER AND WAIST SLIMMER

This exercise uses both sets of oblique abdominal muscles.

Lie on the floor, knees bent up high, and your arms by your sides. Pull in your tummy firmly and hold it there. Blow out and stretch your right hand towards your left foot, twisting at the waist. Hold this position for four counts and then lower back again. Repeat with your left hand stretching towards your right foot. You will not be able to reach your foot at first, but gradually you will get closer. Start with six on each side, and increase to twenty.

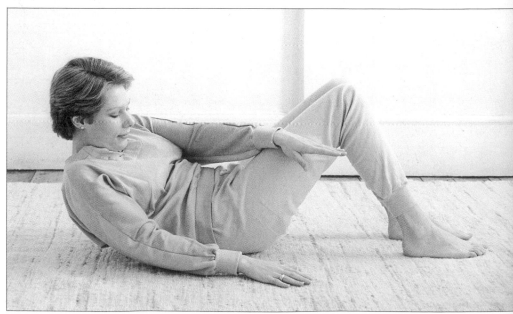

SIDE-BENDER

This exercise will help flatten your tummy and slim your waist.

Lie on your back with your knees bent up high. Pull your abdomen in firmly and hold it there. Blow out and slide your right hand down towards your right foot, side-bending from your waist. Hold this position for four counts, then, still holding in your abdomen, come back to the starting position. Relax, then repeat to the left. Start with six and increase to twenty.

It is most important to make sure that you continue holding in your abdomen during the movements. This exercise can be progressed by omitting the pause between bending to the right and left, and making the movement continuous and faster.

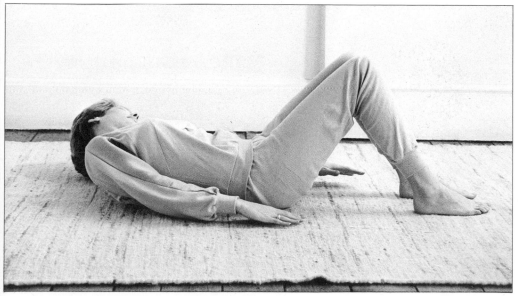

THIGH AND HIP FIRMER

Lie on your right side, resting your head on your right hand with your left hand on the floor in front of you. Pull your abdominal muscles in firmly and hold them there. Lift your left leg straight up sideways as high as you can, without letting it stray forwards or backwards. Hold it there for four counts and then lower. Repeat, lying on your left side. Do this six times each side, increasing to twenty. This exercise can be progressed by holding your leg in the air for longer, up to ten counts.

BUTTOCK FIRMER AND BACK STRENGTHENER

This exercise tightens and strengthens your buttocks and lower back muscles.

Lie on your front and rest your head on your hands. Pull your buttocks tightly together and then lift both straight legs, knees pressed tightly together, as high as you can off the floor. Hold for four counts and lower slowly. Start with six and increase to twenty-four. Remember to breathe normally. If you experience back pain during or after this exercise, leave it out; but continue doing the Back and Buttock Toner (page 57).

SITTING ON THE FLOOR

THE 'DOWNCURLER'

This works your straight abdominal muscles hard.

Sit up straight with your knees bent and both arms stretched out in front of you. Tilt up your pubic bone by holding your abdominal and buttock muscles in firmly. Keeping your back rounded, blow out and curl your body downwards towards the floor. When you reach half way, stop and hold this position for four counts, breathing normally, then slowly sit up. Start with six and increase to twenty.

To progress this exercise, hold the 'down-curled' position for up to 30 seconds; continue to breathe normally. Progress further by putting your hands behind your head.

BOTTOM WALKING

This exercise strengthens your back, abdominal and thigh muscles, as well as slimming your waist.

Sit on the floor with your back straight and both legs and arms stretched in front of you. 'Walk' forward on your bottom, keeping your abdominal muscles pulled in tightly at the same time. Take eight 'steps' forwards and eight backwards. Remember to keep your back tall and straight and your tummy well pulled in as you move. Start with six sequences and increase to twenty. Your baby may enjoy sitting on your lap while you do this exercise.

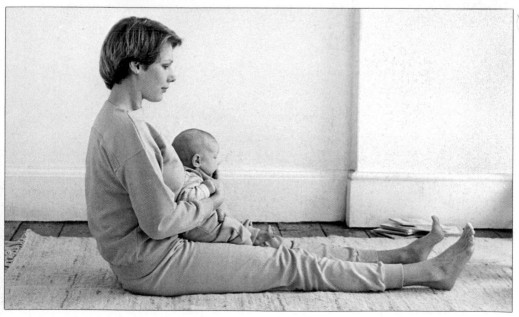

ON ALL FOURS

CAT ARCH

In this exercise you are working your abdominal muscles against gravity. When you are on all fours, you will notice that your tummy really sags when you relax, but when you tighten your muscles to rock your pelvis you can make it quite flat again. This exercise not only strengthens your abdominal muscles but also your buttocks, and it may help to ease an aching back.

Kneel on all fours, with your baby lying on the floor below you so that you can look at one another. Blow out, and arch your back by tucking in your abdominal and buttock muscles so that your pubic bone moves forwards. Hold for four counts, then gently relax your muscles so that your back is flat again. Feel the rocking of your pelvis and the muscles that work to do it. Repeat ten times, increasing to twenty.

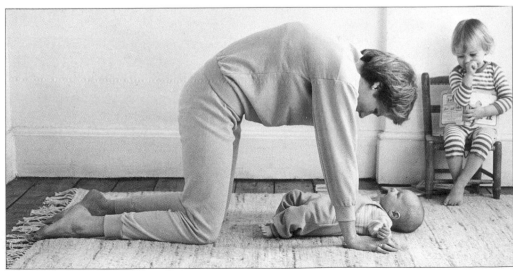

TAIL-WAGGING

This exercise strengthens the abdominal muscles at your front and sides, helping to firm your waistline.

Kneel on all fours as for the previous exercise, with your baby lying beneath you. Pull in your abdominal muscles to flatten your tummy, then turn your head to the right and bend at the waist so that you can see your right hip. Return to the middle, and now turn your head to the left, bending the waist to move your left hip so you can see it. Repeat ten times, increasing to twenty.

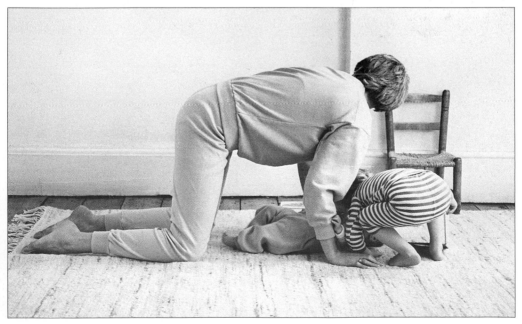

TUMMY AND BACK TONER

This exercise will strengthen the back, abdominal, buttock and thigh muscles.

Kneel comfortably on all fours – your baby may enjoy lying on the floor looking up at your face – now try to touch your right knee with your nose and pull your abdomen well in at the same time. Then stretch this leg out and up behind you, feeling your buttocks tighten as you hold the leg in place for four counts. Lower the leg, and repeat the movement on the other side. To start with, try doing this exercise six times on each side and increase it to ten or twelve times.

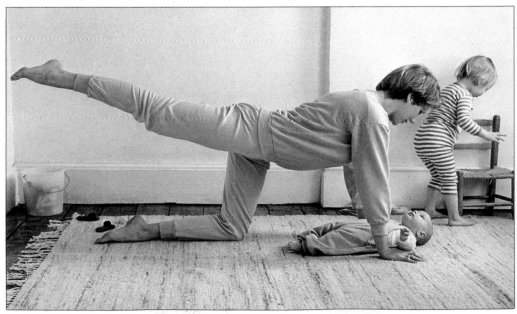

STANDING UP

THIGH FIRMER

This simple exercise strengthens your postural muscles, firms your buttocks and abdomen and shapes your thighs. Do it gently if you have had knee problems and stop if you experience knee pains.

Hold your baby with his back resting on your chest, your forearm lying across one shoulder and his chest and tummy, with your hand supporting him between his legs. Stand with your back against the wall with your feet slightly apart and about 30-38 cm (12-15 in) from the wall.

Pull in your abdominal muscles and squeeze your buttocks together, pressing your waist against the wall. Now, slowly bend your knees and slide 15-30 cm (6-12 in) down the wall, keeping your back firmly pressed against the wall from your waist upwards all the time. Hold this position while you count slowly up to six, then gradually straighten your knees again. As you get stronger you can increase the length of time you keep your knees bent – but not so long that the thigh muscles begin to tremble.

WALL PRESS-UPS

This exercise will strengthen and firm the muscles of your chest and upper arms. It will help you with all the lifting and carrying you will probably be doing by now, but is far less strenuous than regular floor press ups.

Stand with your feet about 60 cm (2 ft) apart. Lean your body weight on your hands, then, keeping your back and legs straight and in line, bend your elbows so that your face is almost touching the wall. Hold for four counts, then straighten your arms and push yourself back. Repeat the exercise ten times at first, gradually increasing it to twenty.

You can work these arm and chest muscles harder by lying face downwards, hands open on the floor just outside your shoulders and pushing your trunk upwards, but, unlike regular floor press-ups, keeping your hips and thighs on the floor. Lower your trunk gently, then repeat slowly, ten times.

DAILY PROGRAMME

Reminder Try to do these exercises the recommended number of times, twice a day. Asterisks mark the most important exercises so on days when you have very little time at least try to do these. Continue to contract your tummy and pelvic floor muscles during feeds.

Lying on the floor

* PELVIC FLOOR AND TUMMY TRIMMER
Abdominal muscles, buttocks, pelvic floor
page 75 6 to 20 times

THE "UP-CURLER"
Vertical abdominal muscles
page 76
6 to 20 times

HIP AND WAIST TRIMMER
Abdominal and lower back muscles page 77
6 to 20 times

* TUMMY FLATTENER AND WAIST SLIMMER
Oblique abdominal muscles page 78
6 to 20 times

* SIDE-BENDER
Oblique and vertical abdominal muscles
page 79
6 to 20 times

THIGH AND HIP FIRMER
Thighs and abdominal muscles
page 80
6 to 20 times

BUTTOCK FIRMER AND BACK STRENGTHENER
Buttocks and lower back muscles
page 81
6 to 24 times

Sitting on the floor

* THE "DOWN-CURLER"
Vertical abdominal muscles
page 82
6 to 20 times

BOTTOM WALKING
Back, abdominal and thigh muscles
page 83
6 to 20 times

On all fours

CAT ARCH
Abdominal muscles, buttocks and backache page 84
10 to 20 times

TAIL-WAGGING
Vertical and oblique abdominal muscles
page 85
10 to 20 times

TUMMY AND BACK TONER
Abdominal, back, buttock and thigh muscles page 86
6 to 12 times

Standing up

THIGH FIRMER
Back muscles, buttocks, abdominal and thigh muscles
page 87
6 to 20 times

WALL PRESS-UPS
Chest, shoulder and upper arm muscles
page 88
10 to 20 times

Post work-out relaxation

Try lying on your back on the floor (see page 43). Relax like this for at least five minutes.

ENCOURAGING MUSCULAR CONTROL

After six weeks a baby's physical development begins to speed up and there are ways you can help enhance this natural progress. Exercises and games with your baby ought to be fun. Remember that they are not a serious activity and should be accompanied by talk and cuddles. Never try them when your baby is hungry, tired or unwell, and stop as soon as he starts to cry for any reason. Make sure that he is comfortably dressed and that his clothes do not restrict activities – ideally he will wear just a nappy and vest if the room is warm and the surface soft. A washable duvet on the floor may be an ideal surface for the exercises as it is firm, soft and clean.

By about eight weeks your baby will have begun to focus and be interested in watching a moving toy; he can usually follow it from one side to just beyond the midline. At the same time the reflex which kept his hands tightly fisted as a new baby is disappearing and he is generally less curled and floppy. In the next few weeks these open hands and more relaxed arms are going to begin exploring his clothes and bedding. He is still unable to hold a rattle for more than a few moments, and it is not until after he has begun to lie and play with his own hands (about twelve weeks onwards) that he will understand the vital relationship between eyes and hands and begin to reach for what he wants. He shows his excitement at seeing a bright toy held in front of him by kicking and waving his arms furiously and he may hit it by chance but is still unable to explore it.

Helping your baby to play

Although he has not yet learned to grasp an object, he is full of yearning to do so. Choose objects that are reasonably large, lightweight and bright, and make a noise when banged, and hang one or two of them over his cot or bouncing cradle (see page 95); he will swipe at them with his arms and occasionally make contact, perhaps producing a noise which draws his attention to what his hands are doing. A large fluffy ball with a bell inside, brightly coloured teething rings, or an aluminium foil plate can be just as absorbing as an expensive commercial cradle game. Once you have engineered the hanging device, perhaps with just a piece of elastic, you can use your ingenuity to think of exciting changes. As long as they are light, have no sharp edges and are fastened securely, then you have an almost endless supply in your own home.

Visual control

By about twelve to sixteen weeks a baby begins to turn his head towards the source of a sound and he can follow a moving object with his eyes from one side over to the other. You can make a game of this activity to help stimulate these vital head and visual movements.

To encourage your baby's visual control, catch his attention so he follows your face with his eyes.

Lay your baby on his back and dangle a bright rattle above him, about 20-30 cm (8-12 in) away, to catch his attention. Slowly move it in an arc, waiting for his eyes and head to follow

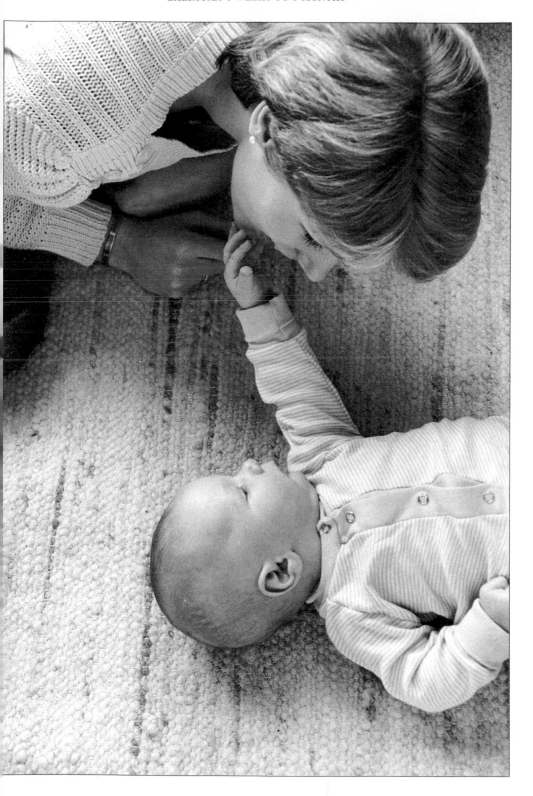

– rattle it to revive his interest if he loses it. Try moving the rattle back to the midline, and beyond it towards the opposite side as well.

Some babies may cooperate in this game far better if it is a familiar face they are required to follow. Try moving your face from the middle to one side, back to the middle and over to the opposite side, talking all the time to keep your baby's attention.

Developing head control

By about two months your baby will be beginning to use his neck muscles to control his head when he is pulled to sitting. You can encourage this important ability by practising it gently with him when he is seated on your lap.

Strengthening front neck muscles

Sit comfortably with your feet raised on a footstool. Lay your baby lengthwise along your thighs, meanwhile talking to him. Put your thumbs into his palms and wrap your fingers around the back of his hands, turning his palms towards one another. Now straighten his elbows and start to lift his head and body gently towards you, talking to him as you do so. Wait a moment and you will see his head begin to lift in line with his shoulders. Pull him slowly up towards you as far as he can manage while keeping his head controlled and in line with his body, and then lower him gently back. This strengthens his neck muscles and

Encourage your baby's development of head control by laying him along your thighs and lifting him slowly towards you while you talk to him.

Babies love to be handled, and tipping your baby gently to one side (making sure his head is always in line with his body) makes a delightful game. Do not tilt so far that his head drops down.

Strengthening side neck muscles

helps him learn to control his head in preparation for sitting.

Another way to stimulate his head control is by tilting him sideways, making sure you allow him time to keep his head in line with his body. Stand with your feet comfortably apart, holding your baby under his arms as you tilt him. Your head and shoulders will tilt also and you can talk to him as he holds this position for a few moments; then slowly return to the middle and tilt him the other way.

By about three months his neck muscles should be able to keep his head steady when he is tilted from side to side. Doing this gently as an exercise will help strengthen these muscles, and your baby will love it, provided he is not tired or hungry.

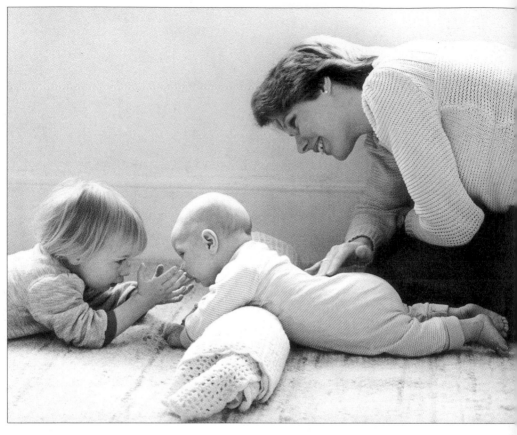

Strengthening your baby's back

It is important for all babies to spend some time lying on their fronts. Placing a rolled towel under your baby's shoulders helps to strengthen his back, while an elder brother or sister may enjoy being involved as well to attract the baby's attention.

By now your baby is probably needing less sleep during the day, and is no longer happy to be put straight back to bed after every feed. When you hold him you will notice he is beginning to look about and that he is getting stronger and can lift his chin off the mattress when lying on his tummy.

Help to strengthen your baby's back with the following exercise. Roll up a clean towel to about eight thicknesses – about 6 cm (2½ in) in diameter – and place it on the floor. Gently lower your baby onto his front so that his forearms rest on the floor and the towel is under his chest. Now talk to him or use a toy to attract his attention so that he lifts his head up. He will begin to work the muscles of his neck and back – some of the muscles he needs to strengthen for sitting – and learn to take weight through his forearms. You may find that gently rubbing or pressing his spine will help stimulate him to lift his head and straighten his back. Repeat this activity several times a day for as long as your baby is happy. If your baby is not used to lying on his front and cries when first put in this position, see if you can distract or soothe him for a few minutes before lifting him up, and try the position again a little later.

Strengthening neck and shoulders

While you are enjoying socializing with your baby, you can also be encouraging him to strengthen the muscles of his neck

While they enjoy each other's smiles, in this rewarding game father can relax while his baby strengthens his neck, arms and back.

and shoulders. Lie comfortably on a sofa with your head propped on an armrest and your baby on your chest. Bring his elbows forward and in so that they lie beneath his shoulders and he can support some weight through his forearms. Talk to him so that he wants to lift his head to look at you and, as he does so, you will feel him pressing down through his elbows and forearms and you can lessen your support accordingly. Repeat this wonderfully friendly activity as often and for as long as you both enjoy it.

Using a bouncing cradle

If you haven't already done so, now is the time you may decide to buy your baby his first 'chair', a bouncing cradle, made of fabric or firm plastic on a cantilevered metal frame. He is well supported in a bouncing cradle and is tilted slightly upwards so that he can watch you while you are busy. You can suspend things of interest in front of him or fix one of the specially designed toys to the frame of the cradle. This type of chair is safe until the baby has started to lift up his head and shoulders, which may be at about five months. While he plays in it, the increasing movements of his arms and legs will gently rock the frame, and that in itself usually delights him even more. It is also light and portable enough for you to take about the house as you move from room to room, but remember that even the smallest rocking motions are enough to move the chair, and it is *never* safe placed unfixed on a table or kitchen worktop.

FIT FOR LIFE

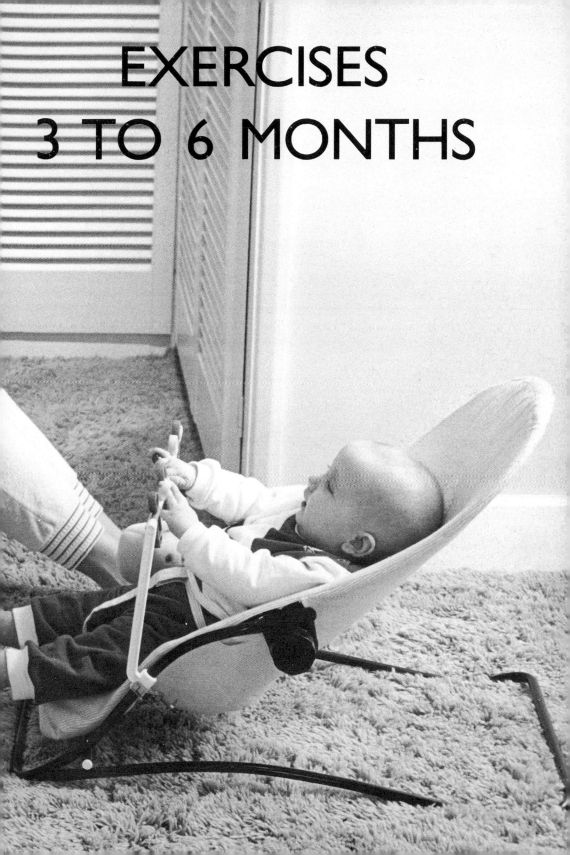

EXERCISES
3 TO 6 MONTHS

If you have been able to do your exercises with some regularity and enthusiasm, your muscles will now be much stronger and firmer and your body will look and feel better than it did. Even if your baby hasn't allowed you time for yourself and you have been unable to do any but the most basic exercises, don't despair, it's never too late to start.

The exercises in this section are very much stronger and will therefore do much more for your figure. If you feel confident about the strength of your muscles, it is perfectly safe to follow the programme exactly. However, if you are uncertain, start slowly and gently – keeping the repetitions to a minimum until you are sure that you are not straining yourself. The test given on page 52 to find your diastasis recti (the gap between the vertical abdominal muscles) will tell you what progress you have made. By now you should find that the gap has nearly closed and that your muscles feel much firmer. (Remember that it is normal for a gap of about 1 cm to persist. The torn strip of fibrous tissue (page 17) does not regenerate, but the strength and function of the abdominal muscles is not affected.) Opposite you will find a strenuous test for that other group of important muscles – the pelvic floor.

Your baby by now will be quite delightful and thoroughly rewarding. Apart from allowing her to join you in your exercises, you will want to use your playtimes with her to help her physical progress in every way. She is rapidly learning to control her head, limbs and body and you will find that very soon she will be rolling and sitting. She will already be communicating her needs and pleasures very clearly and using her voice in various ways. Exercising with her now should be great fun for you both.

Soon you will want to move on from the restricting, and sometimes solitary routine of postnatal exercises and will be wondering when it is safe to resume normal sport. Obviously this will depend enormously on how fit you were just before your baby's birth, and the type of sport you are planning to take up. In the section 'Resuming Normal Exercise' (page 123) there is some basic advice on your choices and the activities best avoided. By the time your baby is six months old you should certainly feel 'Fit for Life!'

PELVIC FLOOR CONTROL

THE ULTIMATE TEST

By the time your baby is six months old you should no longer have any discomfort from your stitches and the strength of your pelvic floor muscles should be back to normal, so that you can control your bladder when you cough, sneeze, or pick up your baby.

The ultimate test for your pelvic floor control is to jump up and down on the spot, eventually trying with your legs apart, coughing at the same time – your pants should stay dry. This does not mean that you can forget your pelvic floor exercises until you have your next baby. Ideally every woman should be aware at all times of this hammock of muscles and the role it plays in her day to day activities and sex life, so continue tightening and relaxing these muscles a few times a day for the rest of your life.

SQUAT TIGHTENING

Squat down, preferably with your heels flat on the floor, holding on to a chair if you find it difficult to balance yourself. If you can't squat with your heels down comfortably try it with shoes on (a small heel sometimes makes all the difference). Your pelvic floor muscles have to work harder in this position than when you are sitting, standing or lying.

Tighten the ring of muscles around your anus, and draw the vaginal muscles inwards and upwards; at the same time, try and feel the contraction of the muscles around your front passage (urethra) too. Hold the muscles braced whilst you count to four and then relax. Repeat twelve times in groups of four. If you find this tiring, do four, rest, and then do another four. Do this exercise three to four times a day.

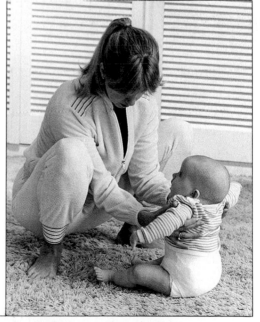

LYING ON THE FLOOR

PELVIC LIFT

This exercise is good for your pelvic floor, buttock and back muscles.

Lie on the floor with your heels resting on a low chair; your baby can lie or sit on your tummy. Tighten your pelvic floor muscles, drawing inwards and upwards; at the same time squeeze your buttocks tightly together and raise your bottom off the floor so that your body is in a straight line from your heels to your head. Hold this position for four counts and then lower. Do it six times and increase to twelve. This exercise can be progressed by holding your bottom in the air for longer – up to ten counts.

CYCLING

This exercise is good for your leg and abdominal muscles.

Lie on your back with your knees bent up to your chest. Blow out and lift your head from the floor. Keeping your left knee pulled up close to you, stretch the right leg out until it is straight and about 15 cm (6 in) from the floor. With a cycling motion, change legs so that your left leg is then stretched out. Repeat for six sequences then bend both knees and lower your feet to the floor. Progress to twenty sequences.

It is vital that you brace your abdominal muscles and make sure that your waist is pressed down firmly on the floor throughout the movement. If your back is arching up as you 'cycle' your legs, it indicates that you are not yet ready for this strong exercise. Concentrate on the less strenuous ones for now.

KNEE ROLLING

This exercise slims the waist and hips.

Lie on your back with your hands behind your head and your legs straight. Holding your knees and feet together, blow out, pull in your tummy, and bend your knees up tightly on to your chest. Keeping your abdominal muscles pulled well in, let your knees roll slowly to the right until your thigh touches the floor. Rest for a moment; then, pulling in your abdominal muscles once again, bring your knees up to the middle. Repeat to the left. Do this sequence six times and increase to twenty-four.

This exercise can be progressed by taking the knees over from side to side without pausing in the middle, and also by increasing the speed of the movement.

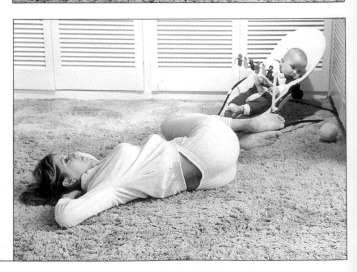

SCISSORS

This exercise tones, shapes and strengthens your thighs and also your abdominal muscles.

Lie on your back with your legs straight. Blow out, pull in your tummy muscles and bend both legs together on to your chest, keeping your back pressed on to the floor. If you are unable to do this yet, slide both feet up to your buttocks and then bend your knees up on to your chest. Now stretch your legs up so that they are at a right angle to your body. Make sure that you keep your back firmly pressed on to the floor throughout this movement. Pulling your abdomen in all the time, open and close your legs, stretching them as wide apart as you can and crossing them first one way and then the other in the middle, like scissors.

Do this eight times, then bend your knees on to your chest and lower your feet back on to the floor, still keeping your back pressed down hard. To make this exercise a little more difficult lift your head. Do this sequence four times to start with, progressing to twelve.

WAIST, HIP AND THIGH TRIMMER

This exercise strengthens abdominal and thigh muscles, and helps to trim a thick waist.

Lie on your side, resting your head on your hand, and balancing yourself with your other hand in front of your body.

Tuck in your tummy and buttocks. Blow out, and lift both legs up sideways; hold for four counts and then lower slowly. Do this six times and then turn on to your other side and repeat. Start with six leg lifts; then progress by increasing to twelve each side.

SITTING ON THE FLOOR

FULL SIT-UPS

This exercise will continue strengthening and tightening your straight abdominal muscles, returning them to full normality.

Sit with your knees bent up high and both arms stretched out in front of you. Blow out, pull in your abdominal muscles and tuck your buttocks under; then slowly curl downwards allowing your back to reach the floor, vertebra by vertebra. Relax. Blow out and pull your abdominal muscles in again, then curl upwards so that you are sitting up straight once more. This exercise can be progressed by omitting the relaxing pause when you reach the floor and then by putting your hands behind your head.

Only begin this very strong exercise when you feel you can really control the movement without collapsing back on to the floor or having to jerk yourself up to begin the up-curl. Start with four and progress to sixteen.

KNEELING UP

KNEELING TWISTS

This firms your thighs, buttocks, waist and pelvic floor.

Kneel up straight on the floor with your arms crossed and lifted in front of you or holding your baby as shown. Remembering to keep your abdominal and buttock muscles firmly pulled in, sit yourself on the floor on your right. Now lift up, holding abdomen and buttocks firmly and adding a pelvic floor 'lift' at the same time, then change to sitting on your left.

Keep the movement controlled, and don't bump your bottom down too hard on the floor – you will not be working the muscles effectively and you may bruise yourself. Start with eight, then progress to sixteen and finally to twenty-four.

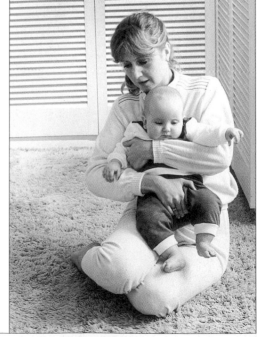

LEANBACKS

This exercise will firm your thighs, buttocks, abdominal muscles and pelvic floor.

Kneel up straight with both arms stretched out in front of you. Tuck your bottom under, your tummy in, and lift your pelvic floor up, blow out and lean back slowly as far as you can. Hold the position for four counts and then return to your starting position. Start with six leanbacks and increase to twenty. You can make this exercise harder by holding your baby in your arms in front of you. Do it in front of a mirror so that your baby will be amused to see you both come and go as you lean back and straighten up (see pages 117-8).

THE FINAL TEST

ELBOW TO KNEE TWISTS

This exercise makes all your abdominal muscles work very powerfully, testing the work you have been putting in to them.

Lie on your back with both knees bent up high and your hands behind your head. Pull in your abdominal muscles firmly, blow out and tuck your chin on to your chest, bringing your left elbow to touch your right knee. Hold for four counts and lower slowly. Repeat to the other side using the opposite elbow and knee. This exercise can be made tougher by holding the elbow-to-knee position for longer, and then by keeping both feet flat on the floor as you come up.

AT THE SWIMMING POOL

WAIST TWISTER

This exercise works the vertical abdominal muscles as you draw your knees to your chest and the diagonal (oblique) abdominal muscles as you twist, trimming your waist.

Stand with your back to the sides of the pool, stretching your arms out along the rail. Pull in your abdominal muscles, and draw your knees up to your chest. Hold the position, keeping your knees pressed together and your abdominal muscles tight, while you twist your knees to the right side as far as you can. Hold while you count to four, return to the middle, and repeat the twisting movement to the left. Now return to the middle and relax. Repeat this complete sequence ten times, increasing to twenty.

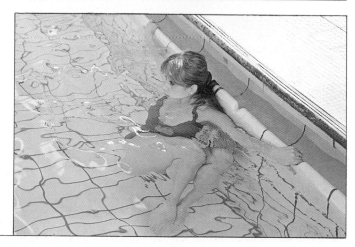

WATER CURL-UPS

This exercise will require your vertical abdominal muscles to work hard against the water's resistance. You will also work your back and buttock muscles to regain and maintain your floating position.

Face the rail at the deep end and hold it with your arms bent and your legs stretched out behind you, so that you are floating. Pull in your abdominal muscles, grip your legs together, and slowly bend your knees up towards your chest. Hold to the count of four, then relax your legs so that they drop down. Now gently kick your legs so that they are once again floating out behind you, and repeat the exercise. Start with ten and increase to twenty times.

WAIST SWING

In this exercise, you are working the muscles at the front and sides of your waist against resistance, hence firming and strengthening them. At the deep end, hold on to the rail with your back to the side of the pool. Let yourself relax with your legs straight and together, then pull in your abdominal muscles and gently swing your body and legs from the waist down – first to the left, keeping your shoulders and upper trunk still, and then to the right. Repeat ten times to each side, increasing to twenty.

DAILY PROGRAMME

Reminder Try to do these exercises the recommended number of times, *twice a day*. Asterisks mark the most important exercises, so on days when you have very little time at least try to do these.

Pelvic floor control

*SQUAT TIGHTENING
Pelvic floor muscles
page 99
12 times

Lying on the floor

PELVIC LIFT
Pelvic floor, buttock and back muscles page 100
6 to 20 times

CYCLING
Leg and abdominal muscles
page 101
6 to 20 times

KNEE ROLLING
Oblique abdominal and lower back muscles
page 102
6 to 20 times

SCISSORS
Thighs and abdominal muscles page 103
4 to 12 times

*WAIST, HIP AND THIGH TRIMMER
Abdominal and thigh muscles
page 105
4 to 12 times

Sitting on the floor

*FULL SIT-UPS
Vertical abdominal muscles page 105
4 to 20 times

Kneeling up

KNEELING TWISTS
Thighs, buttocks, abdominal muscles and pelvic floor muscles page 106
8 to 20 times

LEANBACKS
Thighs, buttocks, abdominal muscles and pelvic floor muscles page 107
6 to 20 times

At the swimming pool

WAIST TWISTER
Vertical and oblique abdominal muscles
page 109 10 to 20 times

WATER CURL-UPS
Vertical abdominal muscles, back and buttock muscles
page 110
10 to 20 times

WAIST SWING
Vertical and oblique abdominal muscles
page 111 10 to 12 times

The final tests

When you can do both these exercises you're ready for anything

*ELBOW TO KNEE TWISTS
All abdominal muscles
page 108   6 to 20 times

THE ULTIMATE PELVIC FLOOR TEST
Pelvic floor muscles page 99
Do once after the first 3 months and occasionally thereafter

Post work-out relaxation

Try lying flat on your back in the yoga 'corpse' position (see page 43). Relax like this for at least five minutes.

112

LEARNING THROUGH PLAY

For babies, the age of three to six months is an intense period of socializing – they are obviously beginning to understand their surroundings, and are just as capable of excitement at the sight of people or toys they like as they are of anger at being denied something they want. Their heads can now move independently but they do not have full control until about five to six months. Although by four months babies can hold their heads up well while sitting, when they are pulled from a lying position their heads still lag behind at the beginning of the movement.

Helping head control

You can help strengthen your baby's neck muscles by practising this exercise every time you pick her up from lying down, provided she is not tired or unhappy. Lay your baby on the carpet and kneel down facing her, with one of your knees positioned between her legs. Move your face close to her and catch her attention by talking to her. Put your thumbs in her palms and wrap your fingers around her hands, then gently pull her arms straight and begin to lift her upwards. Wait for her to co-operate and work her neck, arm and tummy muscles – you will see her head begin to pull into line with her body and feel her arm and tummy muscles helping you pull her up. Reward her with a smile or a cuddle each time she does it.

Propped sitting

Another way of helping develop head control is to prop your baby in a sitting position. By three to four months babies

Once your baby is three months old, with supervision an older child – like this baby's sister – can help to develop your baby's vital head control in preparation for sitting.

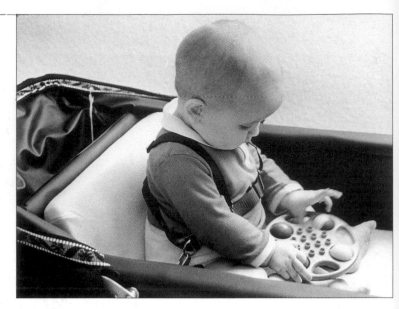

Right: As early as three to four months, you can prop your baby in a pram, lessening the support as her strength and control improve. Even at this stage, however, make sure your baby wears a safety harness.

Opposite: Rolling is your baby's first step to mobility. Start by attracting her attention to one side (top), then encourage her to turn by easing her leg over (below), making sure she does most of the work.

can hold their heads up well enough to enjoy sitting and looking around, their backs being fairly straight, though not yet in the lower part. By five months their heads are even more stable and spines still straighter, and they almost demand to be sat up to watch and play.

If you have a pram it is the ideal place to teach your baby the early skills needed for sitting. Use small cushions or folded blankets to prop behind and to the sides as necessary, and a rolled blanket under her thighs if her bottom slips forward. As her sitting improves, move her further upright and lessen her support, but always harness even a young baby for safety. Loosely suspend some rattles on elastic across the pram so that she can reach for them, but make sure that if she slides down the pram the elastic will not harm her.

Learning to roll

While your baby is learning how to remain erect in preparation for sitting, she is also beginning to learn to twist or rotate her trunk so that she can roll. This movement of the body is necessary for crawling, and later, walking, when the leg of one side will move with the arm of the other. By about five to six months most babies will have learnt to roll from their fronts on to their backs, and by about a month later will be able to roll the other way. You can help your baby roll from an early age when you are changing her nappy – only be careful that you never leave her unattended on a high surface in case she decides she can do it by herself.

Start with your baby on her back, lying on an unrestricted, firm, but comfortable area, for instance, a clean carpet or a blanket on the floor. With your left hand, attract her attention with a bright, noisy rattle about 30 cm (12 in) to the right of her face so that she turns to look at it. Now put your right

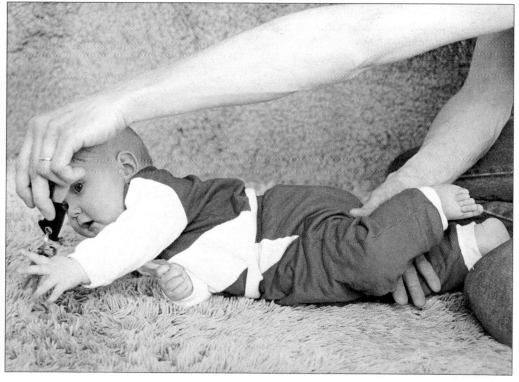

Once your baby discovers her feet, help her gain strength and control of her legs by dangling toys where she can reach them with her toes.

hand behind her left knee, bending it up and pressing the back of your outstretched fingers on to her right thigh to keep it flat. Roll her left hip forward and over towards the right side, waiting for her to follow with her upper trunk and shoulders. When you reverse the movement, tuck her right arm under her chest so that her left shoulder naturally falls backwards. Be careful that you are ready to support her head if she needs it, as the movement in this direction is often rather speedy. Don't forget to roll her in the other direction too. This movement will quickly become natural, and you will be able to decrease your assistance as she learns to rotate her body herself – leading either with an arm or a leg.

Encouraging foot play

At about five months or perhaps a little later, babies have usually begun to learn about their feet by feeling and holding them with their hands, and using them to hit at toys the way they have already learnt to do with their hands. This is an important stage of their development as it teaches them body awareness and how to begin controlling their legs.

You can encourage this skill through play. Try holding your baby's hands while suspending a mobile or 'cradle gym' above her hips, so that she can easily see it. You may need to arouse her interest by touching her foot against it and making it move or rattle. Now wait and see if she takes her own feet back up to it to play with it herself. She will probably enjoy this activity best if she is lying without a nappy on.

Back and arm strengtheners

By about five months babies have enough strength in their backs and arms to take weight on their hands when they lie on their fronts – their straight arms lifting their chests off the floor.

You can exercise and further strengthen these important muscles by encouraging your baby first to look at a toy dangled in front of her face and then above her head, and finally to reach for one, all while she is lying on her front. To start with she will

Right: The mirror game helps to strengthen your baby's back and neck muscles while amusing her with one of the most fascinating people in her life – herself! Make sure the chest support is as little as necessary, to allow her back muscles to work hard (see page 118).

Below: Encourage your baby to push up with straight arms by attracting her attention above her head.

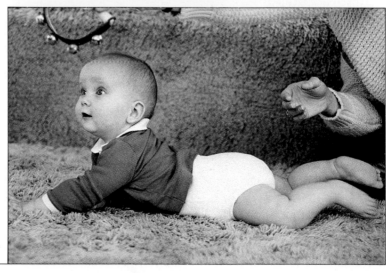

probably only be able to take weight on one straight arm for a brief moment, and reach for a toy on or only just above the ground. As her strength and co-ordination improve you will be able to hold the toy further up in the air so that she has to reach for it – but never allow her to become frustrated and upset by this game. It should be fun for you both.

Neck and back strengthener

You can further strengthen your baby's neck and back muscles by playing with her in front of a mirror. Kneel down holding your baby with her back to you, facing a large mirror. By about five months she will probably like to smile at her own reflection, so give her time to see herself in the mirror before you start. With her feet on your thighs (she will probably enjoy standing on you at this stage), hold one hand in front of her knees and the other supporting her chest, and slowly lower her towards the mirror. Allow her head and back to work as you lower her, giving her minimal support under her chest. She may begin to talk to herself in the mirror. Hold her there as long as she is happy and you are comfortable.

Encouraging your baby to sit

With the increased strength of her back muscles and her strong neck muscles, your baby is now almost ready to sit alone.

When she has begun to learn how to balance, you can try sitting her on the floor between your legs, with a few inches separating her body from your legs. If she still relies on her arms

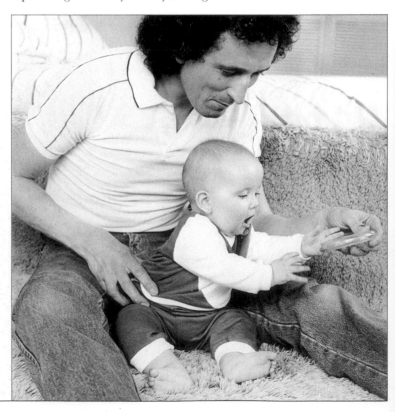

When your baby is almost sitting, play with her on the floor sometimes so that your legs act as cushions. Once she is able to balance without propping on her arms you can encourage her to reach to either side for a toy.

to prop her up in front, try offering her a toy so that she will reach out with one arm. Gradually she will learn to extend her spine even further and sit up without the help of her arms.

Sitting but not yet safe

By about five to six months your baby will possibly be able to sit up without leaning on her arms, but she will probably not yet have learnt the final balance and protective reactions which make sitting alone a stable and safe position. A large cardboard box is the ideal place to put her at this stage; sit her in one corner where the soft sides prevent her falling, and surround her with her favourite toys so she feels safe and secure.

Sitting balance

Once your baby can sit on your knees without support, you can develop her sitting balance further while playing a game. Perhaps to the words of nursery rhymes, like *Ride a Cock Horse* or *This is the Way the Ladies Ride,* you can lift one leg and then the other, starting with small, regular movements, and progressing to larger, less predictable movements, always having your hands free and ready to catch her if she is tipped off balance.

The parachute reaction

From about six months, babies learn to 'save' themselves when pushed forwards while sitting or when lowered head first towards the ground: they react by straightening their arms and putting out their hands to protect their heads. This vital activity is called the parachute reaction and can be learnt and reinforced in play. If you hold your baby at her trunk and lower her, at first very gently, towards a soft surface such as a bed, she will soon

For safety without too much support, let your baby sit and play in a sturdy cardboard box, surrounded by toys.

learn to put her arms out, meanwhile straightening her back and lifting her head. This reaction will be particularly important for her early days of walking when she will fall frequently.

Bath-time swimming

Once your baby begins to enjoy her bath, you may like to allow her an occasional 'swimming lesson'. Run a deep bath and, if you prefer, put inflated arm bands on her upper arms before lowering her into it. Let her kick and splash a little, enjoying the water lapping around her face. Make sure you don't leave her for a second, for obviously she has no sense of self-preservation. It is, and should be, a great game to her, and while she is enjoying herself, she is developing her neck and back muscles but, above all, gaining confidence in the water.

Taking your baby to the swimming pool (see page 122)

After these first 'swimming lessons' in the bath, you can try taking her to a real swimming pool. Once she has completed her first set of immunizations she will be safe to go in the water, provided she is well and the water and air around it warm.

The best way to start is to take your baby into the shallowest part of the pool and just hold her securely, letting her feel the water and absorb her surroundings. Once she is confident, you gently lower her into the pool on her back, supporting her with one open palm under her centre of gravity (probably about waist level), while keeping your other forearm and hand under (but not supporting) her neck and head, in case she tips back. Now let her feel the water lapping around her face and body and enjoy the random movements of her limbs.

Above: Bathtime can be the start of swimming lessons. With one hand supporting her waist, let her kick, splash and blow bubbles. Your free hand is ready to protect her face from accidental immersion.

Once she has good head control at about five or six months, you can start turning her on to her tummy and supporting her

Play and toys

under the chest. She will kick and splash – but watch that she doesn't inhale large amounts of water.

At about three months babies discover their own hands; a few weeks later they learn how to bring them together, to feel objects with them, and to play with rattles which are placed in their hands. By five months they have learnt the vital combination of reaching for and getting the thing they see and want, and they then manipulate it, chew it, bang it and transfer it from hand to hand. By about six months they are sometimes beginning to reach with one hand, and to examine objects very closely on all sides by turning their wrists and hands over.

The toys they need at this stage are few and simple. The first rattle should be one that is bright and attractive, light, well-balanced and easy to hold in a small fist. It should be safe and pleasurable for biting and mouthing, and make a pleasant noise when moved or shaken. The dumb-bell rattle is an ideal choice, as are teething rings. 'Cradle gyms' suspended across cot or pram, and activity boards attached to the rails of the cot are worth investing in to amuse your baby in her cot. Small soft toys are now worth introducing. At this age babies like to bring objects up close to their faces, and small soft toys are ideal because they are safe and easy for babies to manipulate. Babies are wonderfully responsive playmates at this stage, but although you will be finding every new development fascinating, you will probably also be pleased to see how much better they are able to occupy themselves for a few minutes with their favourite toys, a rusk or just a wooden spoon or some paper to crumple. It is really unnecessary to spend a lot of money on toys for a baby of this age.

Baby walkers and bouncers

Although many babies of five to six months enjoy spending time in baby walkers or bouncers, they should not be left in either of these for long periods of the day. The standing ('extensor') phase is only transient and prolonged use of a walker or bouncer can actually inhibit the natural progression beyond it. Babies need to learn to roll, rotate their bodies and move one part or side separately from another as well as simply straightening and pushing with their legs.

Bouncers can cause babies to develop abnormally persistent stiffness of their legs if they remain suspended in them for long periods. At the most, fifteen to twenty minutes in a bouncer at any one time is probably all right, provided the baby has plenty of other opportunities to move freely in other positions.

Cots for the older baby

By now your baby will probably be rapidly outgrowing her first bed and you will be ready to move her into a full-size cot. Modern travel cots may be worth consideration as they are safe, sturdy, collapsible and often cheaper than ordinary cots. However, if you have a back problem, then the conventional drop-side cot will make lifting your baby out much easier and more comfortable. When choosing a drop-side cot, make sure the movable side has a childproof mechanism for releasing it, and that the bars are no more than 6 cm (2½ in) apart.

Transporting the older baby

As your baby approaches six months, you will find she appreciates outings more, and your own movements will be far less restricted or complicated.

Buggies and strollers

The collapsible buggy or stroller is now an almost vital addition to your baby equipment – it is so much lighter and more compact than a pram. Initially you may feel happier if she faces you; as your baby grows you should gradually raise the angle of the seat so that she can look around. She will probably not be able to cope with a buggy in the erect position until she is five to seven months, as she will not have developed the balance reactions in her trunk to keep her upright until then. Remember to choose a buggy which has handles at a comfortable height for you (that is, hip height).

Safety car seats

Babies usually have full head control between five and a half and six and a half months; if their bodies are moved they can keep their heads in line and hold them steady. It is now safe to put your baby in a forward-facing child safety seat secured to the back seat by straps.

When you are are making your choice, make sure that it has been tested and approved by British Standards requirements, and that it has a buckle that is easy for an unrehearsed adult to master in an emergency, yet not so easy that an inquisitive one-year-old can release it herself.

RESUMING NORMAL EXERCISE

If you have been following this exercise programme conscientiously, by now not only will your body have recovered completely from the birth of your baby, but you may in fact be fitter than you were before pregnancy. Now you may want to think about maintaining that fitness through sports or other activities.

Making the right choice

Depending on how fit you were before your baby was born, and how regularly you have done your postnatal exercises, you may be able to introduce other sporting activities before the end of six months. Certainly swimming, walking distances, gentle yoga and cycling can be started by most women much earlier than activities such as jogging, or aerobic, keep-fit and dance classes. Games like tennis and netball, and especially squash, require absolute fitness before you start – they are not safe ways of attaining physical fitness. All exercise should be enjoyable and invigorating and should never be taken to the extremes of exhaustion or pain.

Basic advice

1 Don't exercise following a large meal or after drinking a lot of fluid.
2 Always warm up and slow down gradually before and after vigorous exercise; in cold weather muscles tend to contract and are more easily damaged, therefore make sure you are warmly dressed, especially for outside exercise.
3 Make sure that you have the right equipment for your sport – well-padded training shoes for running and loose, comfortable, absorbent clothing.
4 If you're taking up a new sport, such as running or aerobic classes, obtain really sound professional advice as to technique and local facilities. Beware of the unqualified teacher taking classes that are too large to be able to offer individual advice.
5 Don't push yourself beyond your own exercise tolerance; muscle 'burning', overstretching and joint pain can be damaging and may result in your having to rest during a period of recovery.

Swimming

Swimming is an ideal way of getting fit safely. You can start as soon as you have stopped bleeding, though some women prefer to wait until after their postnatal check at six weeks. The water can provide both assistance (buoyancy removes the weight of gravity on the body) and resistance, so you can strengthen your muscles and mobilize your joints without the jarring stresses of land sports. If you are still overweight, you are in fact more buoyant, and certain exercises can be easier for you (see page 109).

Once your baby is three to six months old, the whole family can swim together. Hold your baby with one hand under her waist, your other arm submerged and ready to support her head, and she will feel confident in the water.

Simply swimming lengths of a pool is excellent exercise – the heart and lungs are working hard to take oxygenated blood to the muscles. Breast stroke is the most leisurely stroke, but it may aggravate backache; unless you keep your head well down in the

123

water you may over-arch your spine. Crawl and backstroke use more energy, and butterfly is only for the fit person. A relaxed way of swimming is on your back, using breast stroke movements of your legs and supporting arm movements.

Specific exercises to be avoided

1 Lying on your back and lifting both straight legs together.
2 Sit-ups from lying flat with legs straight. (Both numbers 1 and 2 involve risk of damage to back or abdominal muscles, and should only be done by athletes in training.)
3 Forced toe touching whether standing or sitting with legs straight. This can overstretch the spine and hamstring muscles if done in a bouncy, uncontrolled way.
4 'Bicycling' by balancing on your neck and shoulders, or rolling your legs back over your head so your toes touch the ground, can strain and damage the neck and upper back unless your body is well prepared.
5 'Bouncing squats' or 'squat thrusts' can damage the knee ligaments and cartilages. It is important to straighten your legs fully between squats.
6 Forcing your thighs apart by sudden pressure with your arms or hands overstretches your tendons and ligaments causing pain, and achieves nothing in terms of fitness. However, if you enjoy the sensation of a good stretch, make sure you allow your soft tissues to lengthen gradually.

Looking forward

Apart from the few warnings given above, exercise should always be fun. If you follow these few simple guidelines, you can safely participate in any form of exercise – even pushing your pram briskly to the shops will not only strengthen your muscles and improve your health, but will also give you a wonderful sense of achievement and well-being. You have now fully recovered from the physical changes of childbirth, and can begin again to enjoy a full and active life.

FURTHER READING

Relaxation

Simple Relaxation, Laura Mitchell, John Murray 1988

General health

Everywoman, Derek Llewellyn-Jones, Faber 1971
Our Bodies Ourselves, Boston Women's Health Book Collective, Penguin 1978

Breastfeeding

The Breastfeeding Book, Máire Messenger, Century Publishing 1982
Breast is Best, Drs Penny and Andrew Stanway, Pan 1978

Postnatal depression

Depression After Childbirth, Dr Katharina Dalton, Oxford University Press 1980
Enjoying Motherhood, Dr Brice Pitt, Sheldon Press 1984
Postnatal Depression, Vivienne Welburn, Fontana 1980
Postnatal Depression, John L. Cox, Churchill Livingston 1986

Childcare

Baby and Child, Penelope Leach, Penguin 1977
Twins, Averil Clegg and Anne Woollet, Century Publishing 1983
A New Life, Dr David Harvey (ed.), Marshall Cavendish Editions 1978
Book of Child Care, Dr Hugh Jolly, George Allen & Unwin 1981
The Good Toy Guide, Toy Libraries Association, obtainable from them (see Useful Addresses)

USEFUL ADDRESSES

Exercise

Association of Chartered Physiotherapists in Obstetrics and Gynaecology (ACPOG), c/o The Chartered Society of Physiotherapy, 14 Bedford Row, London WC1
Australian Physiotherapy Association, 25-27 Kerr Street, Victoria 3065
New Zealand Society of Physiotherapists, PO Box 5198, Lambton Quay, Wellington
The Sports Council, 16 Upper Woburn Place, London WC1 (01-388 1277)
Amateur Swimming Association, Harold Fern House, Derby Square, Loughborough, Leicestershire
Australian and New Zealand readers can contact their local sports centres and sports associations for information

Yoga

Iyengar Yoga Institute, 223A Randolph Avenue, London W9

As well as contacting national organizations, you should find that Adult Education Centres offer classes with qualified tuition

Postnatal support

National Childbirth Trust (NCT), 9 Queensborough Terrace, London W2 (01-221 3833) – Breastfeeding problems and postnatal support, Caesarean section support
La Leche League of Great Britain, PO Box BM 3424, London WC1X 6XX (01-404 5011) – Breastfeeding problems
Caesarean Support Group, 81 Elizabeth, Trumpington, Cambridge Way, Cambridge
The Association for Postnatal Illness, Clare Deltech, 7 Gowan Avenue, London SW6 6RH
National Council for One Parent Families, 255 Kentish Town Road, London NW5 2LX (01-267 1361)
Gingerbread Association for One Parent Families, 35 Wellington Street, London WC2 (01-240 0953)
Parents Anonymous (London) for Distressed Parents, 6 Manor Gardens, London N7
office: (01-263 5672)
lifeline: (01-263 8918)
National Women's Register, National Office: 247 Warwick Road, Solihull, West Midlands (021-7061101)
Childbirth and Parenthood Association of Western Australia, PO Box 230, Subiaco, 6008
The Childbirth Education Society of Australia and New South Wales, PO Box 58, Forestville 2087
The Federation of New Zealand Parents Centre, PO Box 29, 094 Fendalton, Christchurch
Marriage Guidance Council/RELATE, Little Church Street, Rugby, Warwickshire (0788-73241)
For local branches see Telephone Directory
MA MA (Meet a Mum Association), 3 Woodside Avenue, South Norwood, London SE25 (01-654 3137)
Family Planning Association National Office, 27 Mortimer Street, London W1 (01-636 7866)
For local clinics see Telephone Directory
Samaritans – 24-hour emergency service, 17 Uxbridge Road, Slough, Berkshire (0753-32713 or Local Directories)

Toys and Supplies

National Toy Libraries Association, 68 Churchway, London NW1 (01-387 9592)
Snugli – Baby Sling: Branches of John Lewis Partnership and National Childbirth Trust
Vogue Pattern for Carrying Sling (like Snugli): Vogue Pattern no 8287 – obtainable from local stockists or Vogue Pattern Service, New Lane, Havant, Hants PO9 2ND

INDEX

ACKNOWLEDGMENTS

Authors' acknowledgments

The authors would like to thank:
Professor Murdoch Elder and all the
midwives at the Hammersmith Hospital,
London, for their advice and for allowing
us to make use of the hospital facilities;
Jill Hens, District Dietician at St Mary's
Hospital, London, for her professional
advice; Nicky Adamson, Pippa
Rubinstein, Caroline Hillier and Sandra
Lousada for their guidance, support and
creativity; and especially our husbands,
Iain and Martin.

Publishers' acknowledgments

The publishers would like to thank the
following families for allowing themselves
to be photographed for this book: Julie,
Paul and Adèle Cronin; Lucinda, Henry,
Clare and Nicholas Zarb; Linda, Tom,
Tania and Katie Davies; Joanna and
Ruth Pambakian; Frances and Jesse
Parker; and all the mothers at the
Hammersmith Hospital postnatal exercise
classes.

The Ajanta rug was kindly supplied by
Habitat Designs Ltd.

Illustrations

Anatomical illustrations by Elaine
Anderson Figure illustrations by Howard
Pemberton Daily programme figure
illustrations by Russell Barnett

Revisions editor Barbara Vesey

Editor Nicky Adamson
Art editor Caroline Hillier
Designer Anne Fisher
Series editor Pippa Rubinstein

Art director Debbie MacKinnon

Typeset by Media Typesetting
& Productions Ltd, Hong Kong
Origination by Newsele s.r.l., Milan